I'LL SEE YOU LATER

Jack —
To a fellow thespian —
Sure glad we met in Florida
land — great times !
Always have fun !
Cathie Higgins Dow

I'LL SEE YOU LATER

Cathie Higgins Weir

Edited by: Wilma Kahn
                     Leeanne Seaver
                     Deb Hanley
                     Bev Riley
                     Laura B. Willbur
                     Kitty Kachniewicz
                     Glyni Fenn
                     Kathleen Weissert

Book Cover Design by Cathie Higgins Weir

ISBN-13: 9781979137386
ISBN-10: 1979137382

Second printing March 2018.

I dedicate this book to my husband,
RICH WEIR

The course of true love never did run smooth.
William Shakespeare, *A Midsummer Night's Dream*

I'll give you a nickel if you read this one!

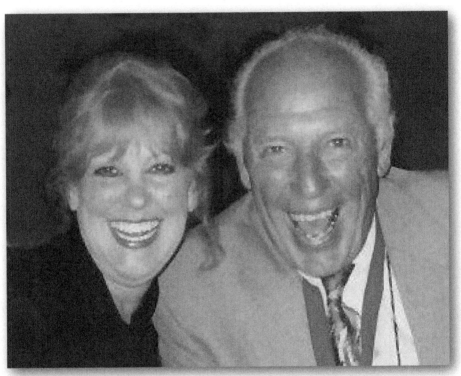

Jim Carver & me Torrington, CT 2003

FOREWORD

By James C. Carver

Cathie Weir is a theater person.

Theatre people are storytellers.

They don't just tell us an event happened, they tell us what happened in minute detail. The more detail the better. They tell us how it all got started; where the action took place; who was involved; how they felt; what they tried to do; how the event changed relationships; how the event changed their lives; they show the strengths and weaknesses of all the characters; they make us root for the major character fighting against all the opposing forces.

As readers, we align ourselves with our own heroes and we despise our villains. We hope our hero has the strength to overcome adversity. We cry when the story teller expresses sad situations; we cheer when there is a minor victory. What happens in theatre is that we, as listeners, become part of the action. We are thinking the thoughts and feeling the emotions of the characters. We become the character intellectually and emotionally. It's a rollercoaster ride for us: sometimes we can't catch our breath because of the events we are witnessing, and sometimes we can relax as we see things being resolved. But we continue with the story because we must know how it plays out.

You are about to launch into a reading experience you will have to stay with until the "final curtain." It is a story of an experience none of us wants to have, and told with such humor you'll be asking yourself, "Why am I laughing about a situation so dire." On one page, I was thinking "OMG, girl. How did you do it?" And the next page I'm laughing my tail off at the antics of my favorite wingnut, Cathie Higgins Weir. I could not stop reading **I'll See You Later**. It is an emotional rollercoaster from start to finish. Just when you think the curtain is about to drop and you can applaud, you find this is only ACT ONE. There are several more ACTS and no intermission.

But what you need to appreciate, through the duration of this story, is the STRENGTH, LOVE and HOPE.

Having said all that, as grim as it might sound, there is so much humor in the telling of this story. There is only one person in the world who could make jokes about the terrible things she was experiencing. Even the titles of her chapters are chosen for their humor. If you're a theatre person, you'll get the bit. If not, find someone to "'splain it" to you. I love the fact that she chose STEEL MAGNOLIAS for one of the titles, because that's what our Cathie is.

SCENES

Okay, that didn't just happen. It was a dream. Wasn't it? No, that was real. It felt real. The machines churned laboriously. The faint light became dimmer, the dreary walls seemed duller.

He entered the room dressed in his off-the-rack suit from Sears. But wait a minute, something wasn't right. He never dressed up. What was happening?

*He walked over to the bed, gently took my hand. **"I'll see you later,"** my father said. But it wasn't with words . . . telepathically? Even though I saw him, I heard him, I felt him, I knew it couldn't be real. My father had been dead for 37 years.*

He passed away at the age of 59 due to complications from emphysema. When I was diagnosed with the same disease at 56, I was terrified I only had three more years to live.

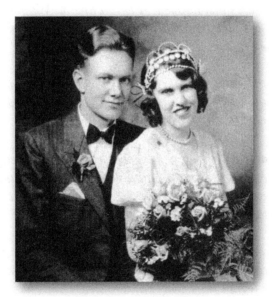

Dad & Mom wedding 1939

Author's Note
ONCE UPON A MATTRESS

*Believe in your dreams. They were
given to you for a reason.*
-KATRINA MAYER

That dream actually happened in October 2007, three months before I underwent a bilateral lung transplant. "Abbey seein' ya" was my father's special way of saying goodbye. So, I wondered why he said, "**I'll See You Later**," but then I realized he had a message for me.

When I tell people about the transplant I'm met with a myriad of reactions. Some people shriek, "OH MY GOD, ARE YOU OKAY?" They are amazed that such a thing exists and are eager to hear my story.

Some individuals ask if I drive. I'm confused as to how a lung transplant would affect my driving ability. Maybe they're surprised that I'm getting out on my own. But driving is not the issue. After parking, walking to my destination is the issue. That's where the handicapped tag comes in handy. I procured mine right after I was diagnosed with emphysema. While waiting in line for my tag,

I recalled a commercial from years before. There was a man with one leg who was standing by a car parked in a handicapped space. The camera zoomed in to show the car's rear view mirror without the designated tag. The camera then zoomed back to the man who pleaded, "Don't put yourself in my place." I thought it was a brilliant message.

To be honest, I didn't drive for the first four months after the operation. I was taking some serious medication, a.k.a. narcotics. When I finally hopped in the car and saw cobwebs on the dashboard, I knew I needed to get out more.

The people who annoyed me the most were the smug ones who just had to say, "You smoked, didn't you?" Well, yes, I did. Even though the coffin nails took my father and I should have known better, I started smoking in the '70s. It was the thing to do to be cool. When I began my career in theatre, everyone smoked so I fit right in. Even when it was discovered how harmful cigarettes could be, I continued smoking. And in my youth, I drank rum and Coke and could roll a joint with the best of them. And yes, I did inhale.

I'm sure smoking amplified my emphysema, but it wasn't the only cause. In 1967 when my father was diagnosed, the tests revealed Alpha 1 Antitrypsin Deficiency[+1], "*a liver producing protein that protects the lungs.*" This condition contributed to his demise, and in 2006 it was a determining factor in my diagnosis as well.

I used to get frustrated with people who had no reaction at all. Just a glazed stare. It was though I told them I did the laundry or shampooed my hair. I wanted to scream at them, DO YOU HAVE ANY IDEA WHAT I'VE BEEN THROUGH? But then I would stop and think, well no, they don't. Why should they? I certainly knew nothing about lung transplants before I had one.

In writing this book I wanted to tell my story, encourage others to let humor guide them through challenging situations or illnesses, to teach people to become their own advocates, and to promote the necessity of organ donation.

Before we delve into this magical medical tour, I'm offering a little background music. So, fasten your seat belts, it's going to be a bumpy ride.

~ Cathie Higgins Weir ~

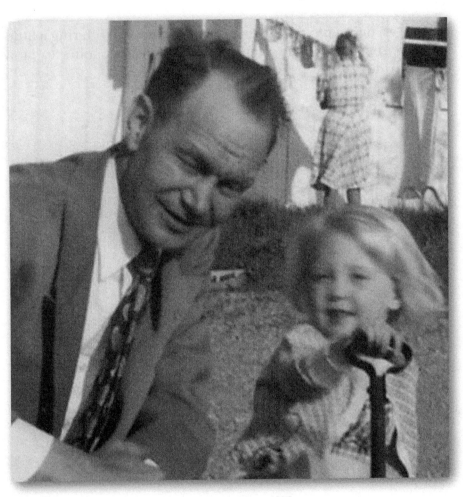

Dad and me circa 1952

Chapter 1

DA

Higgins Hill . . . where anything can happen and usually does. That was the credo of our home in Kalamazoo, Michigan. The door was never locked, and visitors were always welcome. They entered from the breezeway, through to the kitchen, to the dining room, and then into the living room. Everyone stopped by the refrigerator to grab a beer or another beverage on the way in, any time, day or night.

Middle class, hardworking, honest, and respectable folks, my parents, Danford Henry Higgins and Louise Nyoda Stebbins, met at the Kalamazoo State Hospital during the Depression. She was a nurse's aide and he worked in the laundry. Both were extremely lucky to have jobs through those turbulent years. My siblings and I questioned the validity of their claims and teased that maybe, just maybe, they were the mental patients.

Sporting a Cheshire Cat grin, Dad was five feet nine inches tall and skinnier than a rail. If he weighed more than 110 pounds, I would be surprised. Born in Paw Paw, Michigan he grew up on a farm, but in later years he became a house painter/interior designer long before it was fashionable. He was 39 years old when I was born.

His clothes reeked of paint and turpentine, but mostly of cigarettes. At that time, paint was full of lead and he smoked two packs of Lucky Strikes a day. His cough could wake the dead and every-one in the family chastised him for smoking. We loved him and didn't want anything to happen to him.

He loved hunting, fishing, playing cribbage and drinking beer. His nickname was "Splash," referencing an incident where he tried to step out of a boat onto the pier, but in his inebriated condition, he fell into the murky water.

From Chicago, Mom was the typical 1950's mother: house clean-ing, grocery shopping, and cooking, although she would have benefited from Julia Child's culinary lessons. She had a wonder-ful sense of humor. She only had an eighth-grade education, but graduated with high honors from the school of hard knocks.

Mom, at five feet two inches, was defined as "pleasingly plump." After bearing five kids, she was entitled. In the 50's physical fit-ness wasn't as prominent as it is today. As a stay-at-home Mom, she cared for my oldest sister Nyoda who was born mentally challenged, the next oldest sister Rosemary, my brother Larry, and me.

I was 15 years old before I discovered that Mom's first baby, Sally, was stillborn. Thinking about it haunted me for many years. Mom was 40 years old when I was born on May 18, 1950. I was 11 years younger than Nyoda, seven years younger than Rosemary, and six years younger than Larry. I wondered if Sally had lived, would I have been born?

As an adult, I asked my mother if I was a mistake. She hesitated but then said, "You're the best mistake I ever made." I knew it. Whenever she introduced her children, it went like this: "This is our daughter, Rosemary, the nurse. This is our son, Larry, the min-ister, and this, well, this is our baby, Cathie." Maybe my love of the-atre/comedy and all the attention it brought grew out of a need to be noticed.

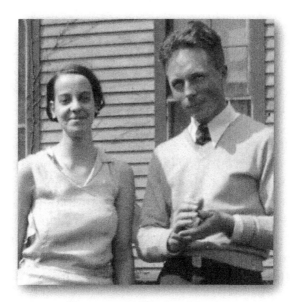

Rosemary & Winslow Martin

Mom was dependent on everyone and, as a result of an unexpected tragedy in her life, she never drove. In 1939, when she was 30 years old, her sister Rosemary was killed when a train struck the car she was driving. My sister, Rosemary, told me how unsettling it was to be named after Mom's dead sister. She explained it this way: *"Any disaster or tragedy was never spoken of in our family. They swept unpleasantness under the carpet, as if it never happened. There were no pictures displayed, or any mementos of our aunt. They wanted me to live up to her memory, but how could I do that when I didn't know what that memory was?"*

I concurred. I had only seen one large photo of my aunt. It wasn't until my grandmother passed away that we discovered a number of photo albums containing unrecognizable people. There were a few photos of Aunt Rosemary, but I was surprised there were no pictures of her wedding. After all, a girl's wedding day is one of the most important days in her life. Why weren't there any remembrances of the occasion? From what little information that was revealed, they approved of her husband Winslow. So why the secrecy?

Aunt Rosemary was not the only mystery in our family. Before I was born, my maternal grandfather, my paternal grandmother and grandfather had all passed away. The personification of mystery was our maternal grandfather. We all have skeletons in our closet, but this was a doozy.

When grandfather Lawrence and grandmother Ethel (Gilmore) Stebbins were married in 1909, mom was six months old . . . an out-and-out scandal for that era. Grandmother was rather plain looking. The only photo we have of Grandpa Stebbins depicts a man who was handsome, dapper and charm seems to jump off the matte photo paper. It was obviously a shotgun wedding, but where did they meet? What could they possibly have had in common? Where did they consummate their relationship?

Another observation my sister Rosemary made was this, *"I never heard Mom say anything about her father. How can you not speak about your father and then years later, name your son after him?"*

The mystery continues with Grandma . . . Aunt Rosemary was born in 1913 in Denver. But in 1918, the three women, grandma, Aunt Rosemary and my mother were living in Chicago with Uncle Franklin, grandma's brother. Grandpa was still in Colorado. Why were they living in different cities? Knowing the circumstances, we siblings assumed he was a dead-beat dad. We didn't have a very high opinion of him.

I discovered Grandpa's obituary in 2017 and learned of another side of his character. I have since reversed my feelings and now feel a sense of pride. In early 1900 when working conditions were atrocious, Grandpa was instrumental in improving the quality of his environment. As a matter of fact, when other family members read the obit, they theorized that his death may not have been accidental.

Note the spelling of the name, Stebenne. Grandmother, however used a different spelling: Stebbins. Just another ambiguity.

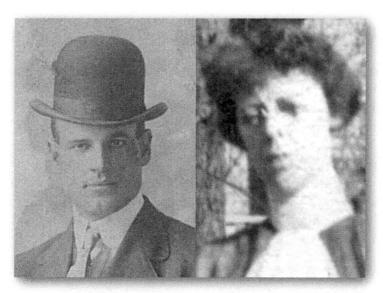

Grandpa and Grandma Stebbins

[2] *On the night, just before he met his death, and after a two-hour session, he was successful in securing the signature of the company to an agreement recognizing the labor union and doing away with the open shop, which had been the policy of the company for many years. Labor lost a valuable member in the death of Larry Stebenne."*

Continuing with the 1950's . . . Mom and Dad were responsible for Grandma Stebbins and provided her with a miniscule apartment on the second floor of our home. Grandma would come downstairs for meals, and even "help" in the kitchen at times. When that happened, the intensifying steam wasn't just from the pots. There was an uneasy tension between those two. We wondered if the hidden tragedies were the cause of their frazzled relationship. With the dishes hand-washed and dried, Grandma would return upstairs to her sanctuary and Mom would go to bed and read. Each to her own corner - only to come out the next day sparring.

Another mysterious character hanging in our family tree is my grandmother's brother Franklin Gilmore who died when I was nine. When he visited us from Chicago, he always arrived in a shiny new car, dressed to the nines complete with a bowler and a gold tipped walking stick. I loved the stories he told about WWI and big city life. I thought he was magnificent.

When they discovered his body, it was revealed that his true persona was significantly opposite from the way he portrayed himself. He had been living in a seedy neighborhood in Chicago among squalor and decay. My parents would have gladly offered him a room, so why did he choose to live in that situation?

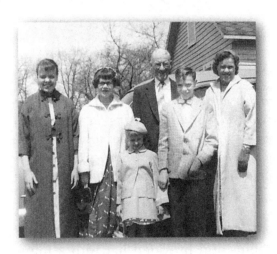

Rosemary, Nyoda, Uncle Franklin, Larry, Mom with me in front. Circa 1955

If you asked each of the Higgins siblings about the kind of home we grew up in, you would receive four different answers. From my perspective, our parents were supportive of any endeavor, no matter how frivolous. They believed we could do whatever we wanted if we put our nose to the grindstone. They were proud of our accomplishments, attended and participated in all our school functions and were active in, and attended all school functions.

Rosemary and Larry saw it differently. The older three kids, closer in age, were born at a time when my parents had little in the way of money or material possessions. There was a constant battle for attention as well as conflict and contention over my grandmother and my sister Nyoda.

The best word to describe Nyoda would be exuberant. She had the embarrassing habit of behaving like an untrained puppy. The minute anyone came through the door she would bowl them over with hugs and kisses. She didn't understand the rule of "don't talk to strangers" and this often created some dicey situations. Our parents didn't discourage her behavior and wanted us to treat her as a "normal" child. They insisted Nyoda be included in whatever Rosemary and Larry were doing. All involved were saddled with a heavy burden, but I was too young to understand their plight.

Recreation was a family affair. We spent most of our holidays with dozens of cousins, aunts, and uncles. Family was important then. It's unfortunate my generation hasn't kept up that tradition. Activities included playing cards and games, birthday parties, family reunions, kick the can, hide and go seek, trips up north, to Saugatuck, our aunt's cottage on Three Mile Lake, swimming, fishing, and for the men, hunting.

My favorite activity with my father was watching *The Twilight Zone*. Our one and only rotary-dial phone with a 15-foot cord was in the breezeway while the TV was in the living room. During one frightening episode, Dad received a call and was gone for what seemed like an eternity. During the commercial when I couldn't stand it anymore, I ran out to the breezeway and begged him to get off the phone to finish watching with me. He did.

We would put on plays in our basement and invite the neighbors over to observe our triumphs. We only charged a nickel. The "scripts" were made up by a collaboration of the kids—lots of fantasy. Much to our mother's dismay, the "costumes" consisted of sheets, towels, and old clothing. We shaped the garments into kings and queens, or so we believed at the time. It was then that I discovered the power of making people laugh. My father was the best audience member. He laughed the hardest and longest at anything we attempted.

All the Higgins' offspring would agree that our parents taught us valuable lessons, especially finding humor in any situation. That's not to say there wasn't discipline when needed. "Wait till your father gets home" was a real threat. They taught us to be respectful of others and set the groundwork for the responsible adults we became.

I was a good little girl and remember being spanked only one time. I was trying to make a slide into my rubber swimming pool, so I used an axe to put notches in one of Dad's favorite trees. The punishment was deserved because a.) it was an AXE and b.) it was his favorite tree.

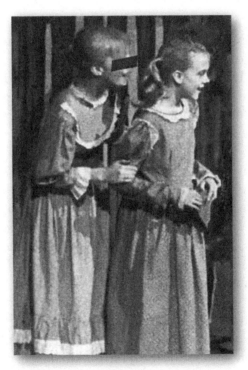

Daniel Boone 1962, I'm on the right

In the fourth grade my teacher recognized my fascination with performing. She sent a letter to my parents encouraging them to enroll me in classes at the Kalamazoo Civic Theatre. They complied, and it was one of the best decisions they ever made on my behalf. Little did I know that the classes would lead me to a lifelong career.

Besides emphysema, another trait I received from my father was Dentinogenesis imperfecta . . . a genetic disorder that causes teeth to be discolored (most often a blue-gray or yellow-brown color) and translucent giving teeth an opalescent sheen. Teeth are also weaker than normal, making them prone to rapid wear, breakage, and loss.

I was skinny, extremely skinny, had decaying teeth and stringy hair. I was teased incessantly because of it. Today they call it bullying. No matter what the name, it is hurtful and leaves scars for a lifetime. Thankfully, I found my voice through the theatre. It was a great education in self-confidence and acceptance, and I thrived in that environment.

In 1957, for reasons unknown to me, Nyoda was placed in the Coldwater State Home[3]. She was among hundreds of people with varying degrees of disabilities, many worse off than she. The kids who disturbed me the most were the beautiful children with big bulbous heads—water head children—I was told. Some had cages around their skulls to support the weight. It was a jolting sight for a seven-year-old girl.

Nyoda would come home for holidays and special occasions. As the years went by, I began to enjoy her company. She loved to tell really bad knock-knock jokes like:

Knock, Knock
Who's there?

Alex.
Alex who?
Alex the questions around here.

Nyoda loved movie stars. Through her Hollywood magazines she learned how to send away for autographed photos. A dozen albums were filled with pictures of her favorites: Red Skelton, Liberace, Roy Rogers, Dale Evans, and countless others. She was rough on her personal possessions and during the many moves to different homes, her albums were lost or destroyed.

By the time I turned 12, Rosemary had gotten married and moved away, Larry had joined the Navy and Grandma went to a nursing home. The constant turmoil subsided, and I was the only child left at home. It was a relief. I had my parents all to myself. By then, they were financially stable, and I reaped the benefits of their good fortune.

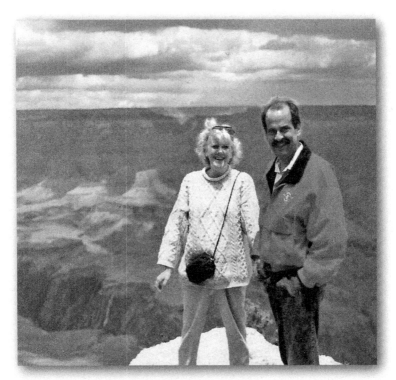

Grand Canyon adventure

Chapter 2
TRUE WEST

After three alarming hospital stays, my father's health was failing, and everything changed. His pulmonologist suggested moving to Arizona, as the air is "cleaner" out there. We had several cousins living in Tempe and Phoenix, so my parents wouldn't be facing the unknown alone. When they decided to heed the doctor's advice they gave me a choice. I could move to Arizona with them, or stay in Kalamazoo with my "steady" boyfriend. I was a senior in high school with only four months before graduation. I was in love—you know, that teenage, hormonal love. It was a grueling decision. I knew in my heart that Dad didn't have long to live, so I chose him.

I wasn't the only sibling affected by this decision. When my parents conveyed to the Coldwater State Home that they were moving, they had to sign away their parental rights to the state. It wasn't long after that Nyoda was shifted from one group home to another. It must have been unsettling for her and heart wrenching for my parents. But I was a teenager, and unfortunately, she was the furthest thing from my mind.

The Muse was with me when I was having difficulty writing about this part of my life. I was looking for a highlighter when I opened a drawer and right on top was a paper I had written in 1968. It was on my father's letterhead, written in my mother's hand with a red pencil. She must have found it in one of my secret hiding places and copied it. When I read it, I didn't recognize the 18-year-old girl who penned it, but all the emotions washed over me again. Even though it was fifty years ago, I'll never forget.

HIGGINS *Decorating Service*

127 **West Cork Street** - Kalamazoo, **Michigan** - Phone 344-7053

WHY

Ever since I've arrived here I've been asking myself why. Why am I here? I don't belong. Why did I give up my happiness for someone else's? Because they are my parents and I feel I owe what I can give them. I missed out on the fun at both schools. Where are the friends I dreamed about? Could I possibly dream up someone like the friends I had back home? I left someone very special in my life; someone who loved me and wanted me more than anything in the whole world. I gave him up for the love and concern of my parents. It's true I'm here, but what can I do? Go on living my unhappy days? Waiting for a possibility of returning to the one I cherish most? They say we're too young. Are we? Have they shown us what love is? Life goes on and I am caught up in the empty space of it. Longing to return to the boy I love. I can't stand this meaningless life here forever; a lonely life without love. Someday we'll be together forever and my happiness will go on unending. But now? Now is the time to cry.

Seeing how miserable I was, my parents decided that after I graduated I should go back to Kalamazoo and sort things out. A girlfriend offered a room in her home and so it was settled. My boyfriend and I wrote to each other every day vowing our love and devotion. We spoke on the phone, only occasionally because long distance calls were expensive then. Four months passed by slowly and I cried myself to sleep every night.

Finally, after all the waiting, it was here, the last day of school. I donned cap and gown and walked in the graduation processional. After receiving my diploma, I opened it up to discover nothing, zilch, zero, except a note that read, "Check with the office." I was dumbfounded. I knew I had passed all my classes. Okay . . . some just barely. So, I checked and discovered since I only attended four months at the Arizona school, I would receive through the mail, my diploma from Loy Norrix, in Michigan. I contacted the school and told them to save a stamp as I would be there to pick it up.

My "Glad-You-Graduated" gift was a plane ticket back to Kalamazoo. I was so happy. When I stepped off the plane and saw him standing there and all of the love clichés in the world wouldn't have been enough . . . cue orchestra replete with violins.

When I arrived at the high school office I received one more surprise. Earlier in the school year, a hat and gown had been ordered for me. This meant I could walk with the Loy Norrix 1968 graduating class at Western Michigan University's Fieldhouse. I don't know anyone who has walked in two separate high school graduation ceremonies. My parents thought it was a hoot.

About two weeks after being back and dating my guy, I began to feel something wasn't right. Little signs that piqued my teenage-woman's intuition. One night we went to a "lover's lane." When he finished parking the car he started crying. He confessed he had been dating other girls, even my best friend's sister, AND he wanted to continue dating. It was like someone had whacked me in the stomach with a 2 x 4. I couldn't believe it. I argued about all the letters we exchanged with declarations of love . . . how I came back to Kalamazoo just to be with him. Again, with the teenage hormones. He said we could still date, but he didn't want to be tied down to one person. Ultimately, I agreed, thinking that after he played the field he would come back to me. I sat around waiting for his calls which became less frequent. When we did go out, I would find remnants of the last girl he dated, a hairbrush, a lipstick, etc., in his car. I wondered if he was leaving them on purpose. I couldn't stand the debilitating ache in my heart. After a couple of months, I told him I was going back to Arizona, hoping he would come to his senses. He didn't.

I flew back to Arizona in a devastated trance, physically ill. I didn't know what I was going to do. I had all of these plans to be with him, and now those dreams were shattered. I didn't have anything to look forward to. No goals. No ambitions. I felt completely dead inside.

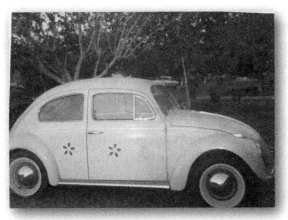

My 1962 VW Bug with hippy flowers.

When I decided to enroll at Mesa Community College, my parents purchased a 1962 VW Bug for my use. The college was six miles away and public transportation was not available. I majored in fashion design with a minor in English. I started dating some nice boys, but I was just going through the motions.

My parents came up with the idea and the funding to register me for modeling classes. It helped break my funk and it was fun learning how to walk, stand, and pose like a model. Twiggy was all the rage and since I was so skinny I embraced her style down to the makeup. The company had a couple of runway shows and I displayed my own creations. When I think about it now, I cringe at my fashion choices. I used a bright red and orange hounds tooth fabric to make bell bottom pants, a vest, and a big beret. Hey, it was 1968.

I started to regain my self-confidence and even picked up some modeling jobs after the class was completed. Close to the end of the session, I went to the modeling school office for something and my folder was sitting on one of the desks. Since no one was around, I sneaked a peek. In my description category an instructor had written "mousey." It was just another blow to my already-shattered ego. I believed there was no hope of ever finding love again, especially if I was "mousey."

After a couple of months, I was hired as a waitress for a pizza parlor. My cousin knew the owner, so I was hired with his recommendation. One of the other duties, besides waitressing, was handling the take-out calls. The male staff would then drive the company car to complete the orders. It was a busy place as Tempe is home to Arizona State University. That job turned my life around and it was the best medicine to cure my melancholy. I made new friends. We all enjoyed working together and we laughed a lot. However, it was Arizona and the pizza joint was HOT and stifling.

A boy from one of the dorms ordered pizzas on a weekly basis, sometimes twice a week. It seemed whenever he called, business was slow, so I was able to talk to him. He had a deep resonant voice, a quirky sense of humor, similar to mine, and an engaging laugh. This "mating dance" went on for several months. One night I boldly asked him, "Why don't you come in sometime?" He told me he didn't have a car plus many other excuses, so I just wrote him off. I was dating two other guys at the time, but neither one rocked my world.

After one slow night, when the boss was out of town and just before closing, someone got the scathingly brilliant idea to have a flour fight. After working in the hot greasy kitchen all night, the flour stuck to our hair and our navy blue uniform skirts had white fluffy hand prints on them. Of course, the girls got the brunt of the attack. My hair was pulled back into a stringy, greasy ponytail. Needless to say, I was not the model I portrayed during the day.

Two customers, male college students, came walking in right about then and we straightened up immediately. One guy had on a camouflage jacket, jeans, and cowboy boots. He had a gorgeous smile, dimples, and beautiful dark brown hair that just touched his ears. I wasn't crazy about the boots, but the rest of the package was neatly wrapped. Without warning, a voice popped in my head: *I'm going to marry that man.* In a split second I jumped back to reality. Where the hell did that come from?

I asked for their orders and when he said his name was Rich Weir I nearly fainted. "Oh my God, you're the face that goes with the voice." Then I apologized profusely for how I looked and explained about the flour fight. He and his roommate were clearly amused. They finished their pizza and left. I felt a connection to him I couldn't explain. For the next couple of months, I didn't hear from him and I figured I hadn't made a very good impression. We didn't exchange phone numbers, but I knew where to find him.

One night, out of the blue he showed up. The two guys I had been dating were both there when he walked in. The way the place was situated, I was able to place all three in different sections, so none of them could see each other. I panicked and was running around the place like a rabid dog. When I didn't hear from him, I wasn't surprised. He was the only one I was interested in and I hoped I hadn't ruined my chances.

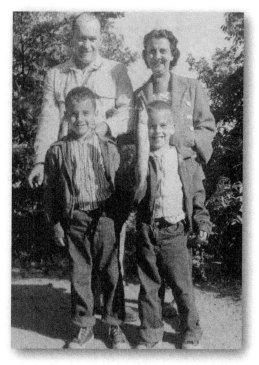

Robert & Delores Weir, Bobby & Rich circa 1957

Months went by and one slow night my friend and I were sitting in the boss's office. The phone rang. She answered it and started taking the order. When she wrote WEIR on the form I gasped and yanked the handset out of her fingers. "When are you coming in again?" He answered with the same excuses. Taking a bold leap, I asked him, "So when are we going out?" He said he didn't have a car. "I do," I said. "How about Friday night? I'll pick you up in front of the dorm. What do you like to eat?" He was completely thrown off guard. Stuttering, he finally answered, "Steak." I told him I knew just the place. So, Friday night came and I picked him up in my white VW Bug with the hippy flowers on the sides. He wasn't impressed with the car, but I chided, "At least I have one." He was all dressed up in a suit and tie. Okay, he was hot in the jeans and camouflage jacket, but in a suit . . . be still my heart. I had on a pretty dress with a designer scarf. I cleaned up nicely as well.

From Tempe, the 26-mile panoramic drive up McDowell Mountain to Pinnacle Peak Patio was, and still is, more than stunning. It was a cool crisp evening. Scottsdale was illuminated in all its glory and the sweet smell of orange blossoms permeated the air.

The restaurant, which is no longer in operation, was a southwest barbeque style where everything was cooked outside. It was a favorite of my parents and cousins and I knew the food would be great. Even though the view was hypnotizing, he nervously kept asking where we were going. He perked up though when within two miles of the restaurant the aroma of grilled steaks overpowered the orange blossoms.

Pinnacle Peak Patio had a casual atmosphere—no ties allowed. When we arrived, the host came at him with a sharp pair of scissors. I shrieked, "Oh no, I forgot. Quick, take off your tie." I pointed to the thousands of ties with business cards attached that were hanging from the rafters. He confessed much later he had just purchased the tie for $20, (that was expensive considering you could buy an entire suit for $25.95 in those days.) Luckily the tie was saved, but I worried how the date would go after that faux pas.

As the date progressed, we were surprised to learn how much we had in common. He and his parents, Robert Grant and Delores Josephine (Alvarez) Weir, and his brother, Robert, were from Chicago. So were my mother, grandmother, and great grandmother. When he stated his grandparents had owned a cottage in Saugatuck, (near Lake Michigan), and were buried there, I practically fell off my chair. As a kid, it was my favorite vacation spot in the whole world.

Saugatuck is a quaint tourist town about forty-five minutes' drive from Kalamazoo. My family visited many times during the summer.

With this commonality, we surmised we could have been there at the same time.

As we continued talking, our shared interests kept mounting and the date went swimmingly. On our second date, he presented me with a huge rose in a brandy snifter and confessed he <u>was</u> impressed with the way I looked on our first date and apologized for the comment about my car. Okay, he's a keeper, I thought.

Further dates included visits to art museums, tubing down the Salt River, and drive-in movies were a favorite. Sometimes we actually watched the movie. We would go out for lunches and dinners. My parents would only go to restaurants for special occasions, so dining out was a real treat for me. I was a finicky eater, but when he introduced me to foods I'd never heard of, I became a "foodie." Being from Chicago, he opened up a whole new world of cuisine, class and sophistication.

We became close, real close and one morning when I woke up, I ran to the bathroom to hug the porcelain god. Oh boy, I thought. How did that happen? We only "did it" one time. I was the girl who wasn't that kind of girl, but I was in love. I made an appointment with a doctor and was devastated when he said, "You're pregnant." I drove up to Camelback Mountain, parked the car, got out and sat up there for a long time contemplating how I was going to tell my parents, especially my father.

How was Rich going to react? And how was he going to tell his parents? It wasn't going to be a pleasant discussion, either way. We were nineteen years old, neither one of us had finished college, and it was just before abortion was fully legalized. The choices I had to make were unsettling. I was sure that Rich loved me, and I knew I loved him and wanted to be with him forever. I couldn't imagine it any other way. Yes, there was a lot of conflict, but I was happy. Scared, but happy.

Rich was surprised by the news, and not especially thrilled. But he put a comedic spin on it when he said, "At least we know we're fertile."

My parents were devastated. In fact, it was the only time in my life my father said something that cut me to the core. *"He'll never marry you,"* he said. It was quite a blow at first, but after a couple of days, I forgave him. He and my Mom both adored Rich and had always wanted the best for me. I understood Dad's disappointment. Because of his illness, his thought process was affected by some intense medication. He couldn't see how happy I was.

Rich's parents, especially his mother, were extremely disapproving. They thought I had ruined his future, but in hindsight it was the best thing for both us. It was a tough situation at the time, but with our sense of hope and humor, we made it through.

While I was pregnant, a funny incident happened at Hobo Joe's, one of our favorite breakfast spots. They had numerous specials for poor college students. Rich mentioned he would like to have one of their mugs. I hope the statute of limitations is over since it's been forty-seven years and Hobo Joes' doesn't exist anymore, but you do dumb things when you are young and in love. After receiving the check, I grabbed one and stuck it down my pants. I figured no one could tell the difference because I was pregnant. As we were walking out the door, the mug started slipping down my leg. I bent over, grabbed it, and my belly, and began moaning "the baby's coming, the baby's coming." The couple with us didn't know what was happening. When we got in the car, I reached up my pant leg and pulled out the infamous mug and we all burst out laughing. We still own that "hot" mug.

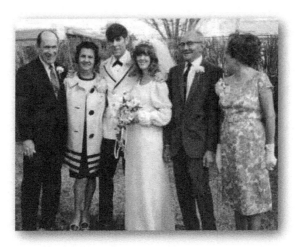

Wedding day: 2/14/70 - Rich's parents, us, my parents

Everything with our parents was resolved and we were married on February 14, 1970, Valentine's Day. You've heard of *Design on a Dime?* Our celebration was "A Wedding on a Nickel." Okay, that's a slight exaggeration, but it was done as inexpensively as possible. In 1968, Franco Zeffirelli's *Romeo and Juliet* was one of the major romance movies of the decade and one of my favorites. Following a McCall's pattern, I made my wedding dress emulating the style of that film. The minister was a friend of my father's, so he didn't charge anything. We held it in our back yard with free chairs from a local church. My cousins held the reception at their home, and my aunt made our wedding cake. I think Rich's wedding ring cost $22 and mine was $19. We have never replaced those rings.

While searching for photos for this book I was flabbergasted to discover a picture of me at four months old. On the back, in my mother's handwriting, was the date the photo was taken: August 27, 1950. RICH'S BIRTHDAY.

Thirty years after we were married, my niece jumped into the genealogy pool with both feet. She discovered that Rich's paternal great-grandfather, who lived in Chicago, was a notions salesman and a milliner. And this is where it gets weird . . . my maternal great-grandmother lived three blocks from his great grandfather, AND she was a dressmaker. I think it's correct to assume they knew and probably did business with each other. With all of the mystical occurrences in my life, I'd like to believe our grandparents had a hand in introducing us. What do you think?

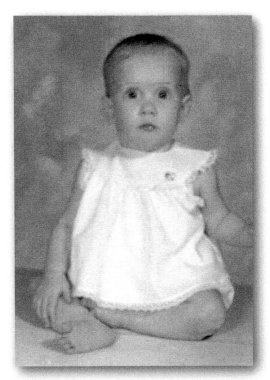

At 6 months, Susan's nickname was Big Blue Marbles

Chapter 3
BILOXI BLUES

In the first few years of marriage, we were so poor . . .

How poor were you?

We were so poor; the squirrels threw nuts at us.

Our only option for a living wage was for Rich to join the Air Force. Not only would this provide a steady income, but the military would pay for all maternity expenses. We certainly didn't have the resources for hospital bills. There was a great deal of apprehension in this decision. The Vietnam War was in full swing and we didn't know if he would be "invited" to go.

The day Rich was to leave for basic training at Lackland Air Force Base, I took him to the airport. He only had twenty-eight cents in his pocket. As he headed for the jet bridge, I shouted, "WAIT." I needed twenty-five cents to get out of the parking lot. So, at nineteen years old, he was propelled into an unfamiliar world with three cents to his name.

Our daughter, Susan, was born on July 10, 1970. I found out, after the fact, that my father had written a letter to the Red Cross asking if Rich could be granted a special leave. His contention was that he and my mother were unable to care for me in the weeks following the birth. Once again, God smiled on us and Rich was able to come home, but just for a short stay.

When he walked into my hospital room, I didn't recognize him. His beautiful hair was all shaved off and he was adorned in his dress blues. It was only when he smiled that I screamed, "Oh my God." I was holding Susan and when he took our baby in his arms, she smiled a great big smile. He was excited about that, but I broke his bubble by saying, " it was only gas."

Now when I look at the beautiful woman our daughter has become, I know someone up there, was guiding us to make the right decision.

When Susan was nine she was helping me with the dishes. Out of the blue she asked, "Mom, how come it only took five months for me to be born?" Oh no, I thought. Here we go . . . the sex talk that every parent dreads. I needed to tell her the truth, so I said, "How about if I was four months pregnant when your dad and I were married?" I held my breath and expected the worst. She let out a huge harrumph and said, "Oh Mom, couldn't you have waited?" And with that she hopped, skipped, and jumped off to her room to play. That's our Susan.

When Rich was assigned to Biloxi, Mississippi, for his training in Air Traffic Control, he went ahead to find us a home. I followed later traveling by bus. Barely scraping by on his income, we lived in an 8' by 40' mobile home. We didn't have a car, a phone, or a TV. For the first three months of her life, Susan slept in a dresser drawer. Someone finally told us we could get anything we needed, free of charge, at Base Services. We found a ride over there and picked out a bassinet and other household supplies.

The "Mobile Home Estates" was about five miles from the base and Rich had to get up every day at four in the morning to walk there. When he came home, he was soaking in sweat and exhausted from the day.

We lived on a diet of bologna, Tuna Helper, eggs, hot dogs—anything cheap. One Sunday we decided to splurge and have chicken and potatoes. We put them in the oven and sat down for a few games of Cribbage. When an hour had passed, and with our mouths watering, we discovered the oven door was stone cold. We had run out of fuel. It was Sunday so no chance of getting any that day. Rich says we ate the half-done chicken. I know I ate the hard potato, but I don't think I could have stomached the chicken. When I watch today's house-hunting and renovation TV shows where the 20-30 somethings walk in and immediately want to redo everything, I flinch. "Get rid of the popcorn ceilings, update the cabinets, and, of course, we need a $3,000 backsplash and marble countertops." I want to scream, "YOU HAVEN'T SUFFERED ENOUGH."

I'm trying to remember what I did all day besides taking care of Susan, but it escapes me now. I know doing the laundry was unpleasant. I took the baby buggy, complete with Susan and the clothes and walked down the dusty drive to the dingy, smelly laundromat. And as the laundromat was not air conditioned, the sweat spewed out every pore in my body.

We couldn't go to the beach as it was off-limits because of residual damage from Hurricane Camille. [4] We were there less than a year after the storm had ravaged the area, and the devastation was still prevalent. When I was able to find a ride in to town, it was eerie to see remnants of the massive, multi-columned mansions draped in cobwebs and Spanish moss. The plays of Mississippi native, Tennessee Williams, came to mind: *A Streetcar Named Desire,* and *Cat on a Hot Tin Roof.* The plays explore themes of steamy, sultry disintegration. The narratives have a facade of southern charm, but the reality is stark, and so it was with these decaying estates.

On November 3, 1970, about two in the afternoon, there was a knock on the door. I didn't know anyone, so I was a little apprehensive to answer. I peeked out the window and there was a tall, frail black man in a dirty work shirt and even dirtier pants. I recognized him as one of our maintenance men, so I cracked opened the door. He mumbled something in a thick Southern drawl, so thick, I couldn't understand what he was saying. He finally blurted out, "Yo daddy's deat." I still wasn't sure what he had said. The look on my face must have prompted him to repeat it. "Yo daddy's deat. You come to de office to call your mama." My daddy's dead? I silently nodded and closed the door. The emphysema finally claimed him. *

*In October of 2016 I took a writing class at a local senior center. It was encouraging to read my material and receive both positive and constructive feedback. In November of that same year, Rich and I, Susan, her beau Aaron, and our granddaughter Hannah travelled to St. Martin for Thanksgiving. I brought along this manuscript to do some more writing. I was reading the notes our instructor had given me. After the line, "I silently nodded and closed the door," she had written, "You might add a little context. Had he been in poor health? etc." I took her advice, thought about it for a while and I finished the sentence with "the emphysema finally claimed him." At that very second, the lights went out and everything went black. Now, granted, they had gone out once before, but at that precise time? At that very nanosecond? Dad was letting me know he's still with me.

Stunned, I put Susan in the buggy and walked to the office to make the call. She confirmed what I didn't want to believe . . . I didn't want to hear that my father was dead. Mom told me plane reservations had been arranged so I could come home for the funeral. I barely understood anything she said, trying to process the desolation. After a long silence, I hung up the phone.

I guess the reality of it didn't set in immediately. We were moving the following month to Myrtle Beach, South Carolina. If I went to Kalamazoo, Rich would have to do the remainder of the packing. Granted it wasn't much, but after a stressful day, I hated to dump it on him. He came home that night and when I told him about my dad, we held each other and wept.

Later in bed I was so anxious, I couldn't settle down. I was shaking violently, and my heart was racing. Never having experienced anything like this, I didn't know if it was part of the grieving process or I was having a nervous breakdown. I had to face the fact that my father was gone and shamefully, I did not want to go to the funeral. I was afraid I would make a fool of myself. I finally closed my eyes really tight and I said, "Dad, you know I love you. You know it hurts to know I'll never see your smile again, or hear your wonderful laugh. I hope you will forgive me when I say I don't want to come to the funeral. I'm afraid I'll behave like a blubbering idiot. I do love you with all my heart."

All of a sudden, a warm glow started at my head and moved slowly down my body, diminishing the shaking as it descended. I heard my father's faint whisper, "It's all right." By the time the light reached my toes, I was calmer and more at peace than I had ever been in my life. I slept like a rock.

The next morning, even though I was dreading the day, Susan and I flew from Biloxi to Chicago's O'Hare Airport. When we arrived, and made our way to the Kalamazoo gate, I discovered our flight had, unfortunately, been delayed. The funeral was scheduled for ten the following morning. I didn't know what to do, so I called my Mom. It was determined my sister Rosemary would make the three-hour drive to pick us up.

It was 1970, long before cell phones, so four stressful hours later I phoned to see where she was. They had been trying to page me, but at the gate where we had arrived, not the gate where we were departing.

The snowstorm and icy roads made it impossible for her to make the trip. When the flight to Kalamazoo was cancelled I made arrangements to go on the flight at six the next morning. I called Rich's parents to let them know the situation. His dad didn't like the idea of me being alone at O'Hare with their four-month-old granddaughter. He said he would pick us up, so we went back to their condo and slept for a few hours.

I woke up the next morning at 4:30, we arrived at the airport and boarded the thirty-minute flight to Kalamazoo. About ten minutes into the flight, the pilot announced, in that crackly microphone voice that no one understands, the weather was unsafe, so they had to divert to Detroit. After landing, I called my Mom once again and broke down crying. I had run out of baby supplies, I was exhausted, and Susan was cranky. Someone finally showed me how to get to emergency services in the airport. What a relief. They gave me diapers and formula. Each woman took turns holding Susan, and she settled down. They also made phone calls for me. They were super.

Eventually we headed back to our departure gate. While I was sitting there, with Susan in my arms, a young soldier approached and asked if I was trying to get to Kalamazoo. He said his mother was driving over and he wondered if I would like to ride back with them. By that time the weather and roads had improved. He asked others in the boarding area, and they filled their car with as many as they could. What a hero. After twenty-four hours of traveling, I finally made it home, but I missed the funeral. Coincidence? I think not.

The following day I went alone to the funeral home and was led to a very large room. It was dismal looking and smelled dank and musty. When I walked over to the gurney where Dad was laid out, I felt like I was moving in slow motion. It was distressing to see his lifeless body and not seeing the smile I loved so much. But he appeared to be at peace. "You made this happen, didn't you?" I said. "Good joke, Dad. I love you."

Later that same day I attended the burial service with my family. It was only an observance as the ground was solid ice that November, so they couldn't inter the body. Oddly enough, I didn't cry.

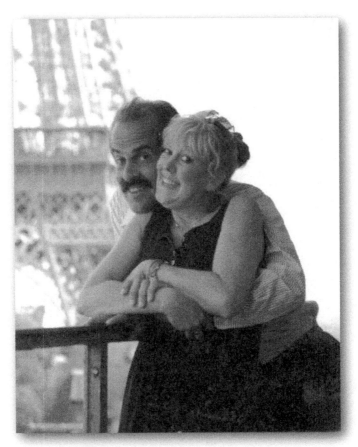

Paris is one of our favorite travel destinations.

Chapter 4
OUR TOWN

Where we lived was determined by Rich's employment, so we moved many times over the years. I would find either a part or full-time job for some extra cash, sometimes as a waitress or an office worker or in retail sales. I'm providing the Reader's Digest version of our various moves, so we can get on to the juicy bits.

1970 - After Biloxi, Rich was one of the lucky ones who received his dream destination of Myrtle Beach Air Force Base, South Carolina. He had attended the Citadel in Charleston, after high school so he was familiar with the area. He especially liked living where fresh sea food was available. We finally had a little money and were able to purchase our first car, a Triumph Spitfire. We also purchased a TV and our parents helped us with telephone costs.

I loved living three blocks from the ocean. It was my main source of entertainment. Susan loved the beach as well, but not the water. When we discovered the base provided childcare services, I landed a job at an upscale boutique as a salesperson and window dresser . . . one of my favorite jobs to date.

1974 - When his four years of military were completed, Rich chose not to re-up, so he could pursue a job with the Federal Aviation Administration (FAA). The Vietnam War was in full swing and we were afraid that if he continued with a military career, it was more than likely he would be heading that way.

We moved back to Kalamazoo and my mother graciously allowed us to stay with her while we waited. Months and months went by and we began to question our decision. Money was tight working for minimum wage at $2 an hour. We worked for Jacobson's, a high-end retail company—Rich at the home store and me at the main store in the men's department.

1975 - After fourteen months, Rich was finally hired for the Melbourne Control Tower in Florida. With another Michigan winter under our belts, we were happy to be moving to warmer climes. We had a lovely townhouse with a pool, so I taught Susan how to swim. She never liked the water before, but when she saw her smaller friends diving off the board, she realized she was missing out. As of this writing she owns lake property and our granddaughter is an excellent swimmer who has won several medals in local and state meets.

1976 - After a year and a half in Melbourne, an FAA job opened in Myrtle Beach. We still had friends there and we liked the area so Rich applied and was hired. Once again, we packed up and moved back to the low country.

1979 - When a job became available for Rich in Kalamazoo, we made the decision to move back to the frozen north. Our parents were getting older and we wanted to be available if they needed any help. When we moved back to Michigan we discovered that Portage schools offered a stronger curriculum than Kalamazoo schools. We wanted Susan to have the best education available, so we rented a condo in Portage.

By this time, I didn't have to work. I had plenty of time on my hands because Susan was in school. I was going stir crazy. Rich knew it when he came home one night. I told him that in the Meow Mix commercial the cats didn't say meow fourteen times but twelve. Yes, it was time to get out of the house!

One Sunday I saw a large ad in the Kalamazoo Gazette for the Civic Theatre. [+5] It was a call for volunteers to fill positions that included set painting, collecting props and stage managing. Because I had enjoyed the theatre as a child, I made an appointment. A time was set for me to meet the volunteer coordinator, a lovely woman named Jackie. When I walked in the stage door the first person I met was not Jackie but James (Jim) Carver, the managing director. At the time I didn't know who he was, but we clicked immediately. It was the beginning of a life-long friendship. After a few months he invited me to do a walk on role in *Don't Drink the Water*. I was thrilled to be making my Mainstage debut with the big cheese, and I do mean cheese, Jim Carver. My love affair with the theatre was born. Through the following years I performed in *Crimes of the Heart, Macbeth, Rumors, I Hate Hamlet, Lettice & Lovage, Annie, The Merry Wives of Windsor, The Shadow Box* and *Outcry*, to name a few.

I think I've mentioned how much I love the Kalamazoo Civic Theatre and how it shaped my life. Well along with theatre, there comes a theatre ghost and ours was no exception. Thelma was her name. No one knows who she was or where she came from, but she was as much a part of the theatre as any volunteer or staff member. Sightings of her report that she was medium height, wearing a trench coat, a hat and carrying bags from the local shops.

Young people involved in Civic Summer Theatre during the 1980's thought she should have a last name, so they christened her Thelma Mertz. I encountered her many times while volunteering, and practically every day I came to work. To get to the office I entered through the stage door, went down a hallway and turned left on to the stage. At 10a.m. the stage was dark with only the "ghost light" showing the way. Every morning I could feel her behind me, and every morning I would say, "Good morning, Thelma," before proceeding upstairs to the office.

During the busiest time of year, the season subscription campaign, I was working late in the office. The heavy steel office door was difficult to open under any circumstances. But that night it slowly opened with a metallic creak. I didn't pay attention because I thought it was someone from the rehearsal taking place downstairs. When no one appeared, I thought, well that's weird, there wasn't any draft. I got up, went to the door and closed it tightly. I sat down to continue my calculations. A couple of minutes later it happened again. Then I felt it. Out of nowhere came a cool breeze causing the proverbial goose bumps. I knew it was her and said, "Okay Thelma. That's enough." I got up, slammed the door and said, "Don't do it again." I would like to say I heard her laughing, but I didn't. The game ended, and I was able to complete my work.

Another incident occurred while I was stage managing *Bedroom Farce*. An integral prop in Act II was a hairbrush. During intermission I placed it on the set in its appropriate place and returned to the stage manager's desk. I never moved from that spot and I was watching either the stage monitor or the stage itself. All of the actors were downstairs, and no one came near the stage until "places" were called. At the moment the actress was to use the brush, it had vanished. Luckily the actress was proficient in improv and made it through the scene. After final bows she had some words with me, but when I explained what happened, she understood. Several cast members help me look for that brush, but even during strike it was never found.

There are stories of a piano playing with no one in the building, a woman's compact flying off a dressing room table, sightings, lights flickering during a séance on stage. You'll find more stories if you Google Kalamazoo Civic ghost stories.

Jumping ahead, I started directing in 1990 when Jim threw a script on my desk and said, "Here. You're directing." The original director had to bow out because of a family emergency. The show was *Eleemosynary*, a play that delves into the relationships between three generations of women. He had encouraged me to direct in the past, but I didn't feel I was ready. I was given a loving nudge from Jim and with the help of many people, it was a success. I went on to direct, (for the Civic), *The Musical Comedy Murders of 1940, The Foreigner, Blithe Spirit, The Woman in Black, Stepping Out, The Odd Couple* (female version), *Sylvia, Little Women,* and *Terra Nova.*

1981 - Rich worked in the Kalamazoo air traffic control tower until Ronald Reagan fired 11,000 Air Traffic Controllers. Rich enjoys saying he was fired by the president. [+6]

1983 - Rich's dad passed away due to complications from Phlebitis. Neither of his parents believed in funerals so his body was donated to science. My relationship with Rich's parents was a constant strain so I don't mention them often in my memoirs. We had been married for thirteen years when his dad passed. I understood why they were disappointed in the beginning, but after all those years, I felt they should have accepted me. I could tolerate their unkind treatment of me, but when they behaved the same way with our daughter, their granddaughter, I put my foot down and said, "enough." Rich loved his parents and it was unfortunate that the visits were so unpleasant.

1984 - I was looking through the newspaper and I saw a job for an Airline Manager. I showed it to Rich thinking it would be perfect for him. He applied and won the job. The company was Simmons which later became American Eagle. With his flying benefits we took our first trip to Hawaii. It instilled a sense of wanderlust in both of us and travelling became an important part of our lives.

1985 - I found myself working in the booking office for the State Theatre. [+7] Local arts groups and city officials, led by Duwain Hunt, formed the "Save the State" committee to preserve the theatre's legacy along with the building. A Vaudeville style show was produced and Donald O' Connor was the guest star. Several actors performed various acts which included comedy, dancing, juggling, and ventriloquism. I did a comedic monologue about *Hamlet* and was next to Mr. O'Connor for the final bow.

1986 - The ultimate thrill of my life was when Jim Carver hired me as his assistant for the Kalamazoo Civic Theatre.

Rich's Mom passed away from Crohn's Disease. Her body was also donated to science. He and his brother flew to Chicago to sort out their childhood apartment. They arranged to have headstones for both parents placed at Fort Custer National Cemetery in Battle Creek, MI.

1988 - When Susan graduated from high school we moved to Kalamazoo making a shorter commute to both of our jobs.

1989 - I started an improvisational murder mystery company called *Suspenders.* I wrote and developed the scripts, hired and fired actors, produced and directed over fifty productions annually around southwestern Michigan, Ohio, and even Chicago.

Community theatre is an all-volunteer operation but with *Suspenders* I was able to pay actor friends a nice salary and have fun in the process.

1996 - Not wanting a full-blown wedding, and with Rich offering some funding, we flew off to Las Vegas for Susan's wedding to Thomas, "Tucker" Rafferty. They had been together for a few years before taking the plunge, so we were happy with the union.

1997 - It was a sad day in the Kalamazoo Civic business office and in the community at large when James Carver retired. He was an icon in the theatre and the loss would be felt for years. Working for him wasn't a job it was a pleasure. He started each day by telling a joke and then he would shout, "Get back to work." He was assured we all knew our jobs, and let us do them without interruption. He was and will always be my favorite boss and mentor.

That same year on July 3rd, I had taken the day off from work because I wasn't feeling well. In the afternoon, I received a phone call from the senior housing complex asking me to come over to discuss some issues with my Mom. I tried to back out of it, but they insisted. When I arrived, there was a flurry of activity in her room. I walked in, saw her, and said, "She's gone, isn't she?" A couple of nurses nodded their heads yes and they left me to wait for the funeral home to claim her body. I called Rich and Susan and they came around 5:00p.m. I called my sister Rosemary, who was out of town. And then waited. It It was a disturbing sight to see them whisking her off in a body bag on a gurney and when the director handed me her wedding rings, I just lost it.

When my nieces and I went to clean out Mom's apartment, we divided up her items. Each of us chose treasured mementos. I went home with a medium sized box to sort. Some to keep, some to throw away and some to donate. I didn't want to do it right away, so it sat in my closet for about two months.

When I finally did take on the task I had another paranormal experience. As I was shifting through the box of memories I found at least twelve cheap plastic combs. I couldn't understand why she had so many because her hair was really thin. I looked up and said, "Geez, Mom, why did you need all of these?" I threw the combs in the trash pile and out they went.

The next morning when I came downstairs, our dog was standing by the buffet and growling. A stray and a mutt, Peanuts was our "he-followed-me-home-can-I-keep-him?" dog. This dog was so laid back you'd think he was on a continual mushroom trip. Since growling was against his nature, I couldn't fathom what was bothering him. I walked over and on top of the buffet was a black comb filled with white hair. I nearly passed out. I just stood there in disbelief. A couple of minutes later, Rich came downstairs. Unnerved, I said, "Did you put this comb here?" I must have looked possessed because he stared at me like I was mad. "What are you talking about?" he replied. "This comb. Did you put it here?" He said, "No, I've never seen it before." When I told him the story he didn't believe me, but I knew it was the truth. When he left I said, "Okay, Mom, I'll keep this one." I put the comb in a photo album where it remains to this day.

1999 – After Carver left the Civic there were interim managers ranging from, (in my opinion), incompetent, to micro manager, to tyrannical, to maniacal. It was so frustrating after working with someone who was so easy. With much anxiety, I felt there was no other choice but to leave. As much as I hated to, it was necessary to maintain my mental health and welfare. I also wanted to pursue my dream of studying theatre in Britain. Shortly after I left my job, I auditioned in Chicago for Atlantic Overtures and was selected to study for two weeks with the Royal National Theatre (RNT) in London. Before the classes started, Rich and I traveled to Ireland for a week and then on to London where we spent one day together. The following morning, he dropped me off at the college where I would be staying, and he flew back home.

There were thirty participants in the program divided into two groups. We each had our own dorm room but shared a bath. The rooms were, as dorm rooms will be, dull. But it was wonderful to have the privacy. The rooms had a single bed, a sink, a closet, a table, two chairs, and a mini refrigerator. I picked up several colorful theatre brochures along with scotch tape and adorned each wall. I even bought two plants which made the room cozier. I stocked the fridge with pâtés, a small baguette, fruits and of course, my drink of preference, Coke. My room was the envy of the floor.

The best part of the experience was two weeks of intensive study from nine a.m. to five p.m. with some of Britain's finest actors, directors and teachers. My favorites were Toby Jones, Selina Cadell, and Sir Richard Eyre, director of the Royal National Theatre, RNT. Sir Richard had worked with the best: Ian McKellan, Judy Dench, and Patrick Stewart to name a few.

During one session, the class was given a backstage tour of the RNT and we were amazed at the posh dressing rooms. After viewing two productions, we were invited for a talk back session with the actors who had just performed. My favorite was Juliet Stevenson. I saw thirteen brilliant plays in two weeks. *The Merchant of Venice* was standing room only, but it was so captivating that the few of us who endured it were amazed how quickly the three hours passed.

We had free time on the weekends, so we could choose what we wanted to do. I took the train by myself to Bath. Rich and I had been there a couple of times before and we loved it. I had a lovely high tea at the Pump Room and then explored the city a little more. I discovered a string quartet in the park and paid £5 for a chair. Sitting in the sun, I enjoyed the works of Vivaldi, my favorite, Bach, Mozart, and Beethoven. The train ride back was standing room only, but I found a place where I could easily sit on the floor by the luggage.

When I learned that Ian McKellan would speak to our group, I was euphoric. He was/is, in my opinion, one of the most brilliant British actors of all time. When he entered the room, there was a collective gasp of enthusiasm. As luck would have it, he sat right next to me. I could hardly contain myself. When he stood up to demonstrate something, he put his hands on my shoulders. I swore I would never wash them for the rest of my life.

Another adventure was when I learned of a military tattoo in King's Cross. No one wanted to go with me. So again, I took the train. As I was sitting there waiting for the event to begin an announcement came over the intercom. "Tonight, ladies and gentlemen, we are privileged that the queen will be joining us," or words to that effect. I could not believe my luck. In a few moments, the arena doors opened, and a brown Rolls Royce circled the stadium and stopped right in front of where I was sitting. I was flabbergasted. Queen Elizabeth and Prince Philip got out of the car and walked right past me. They ended up sitting eight rows behind me to my right. The next day, I had a crick in my neck because I was watching them more than the show.

The opening of the production was one I will never forget as long as I live. There was a massive set of doors at the end of the arena. They reminded me of airplane hangar doors. When the lights dimmed, the doors slowly opened and low-level fog and lighting came pouring out from underneath. Through that fog, fifty bagpipers, in full regalia, marched in their choreographed cadence. It was spectacular.

Later in the program a team of thirty horses and riders played a startling game of chicken. The horses darted in and out galloping at full speed. It was breath-taking. The entire show gave me the chills and at the end of the performance, I was uplifted all the way back to the dorm.

We had a fun group of instructors so the next day, with much enthusiasm, I revealed that, **"I SAW THE QUEEN."** One of them replied, "Yes, I know Sir Ian spoke to your group yesterday."

The classes left an indelible impact on my performing style. So much so that when I performed as Claire in *Outcry*, one of my long-standing friends gave me the best compliment by saying, "Who was that up there?"

With both sets of parents gone, Susan married, and we were approaching fifty, Rich decided to bid on a job for American Airlines in Orlando, Florida. They had great insurance, a quality retirement plan, and we retained our flying benefits. He was hired as a Customer Service Manager, so we were off on another adventure.

Before moving there, I spent hours researching the theatre culture and was excited to learn of all the opportunities available. I had registered for an acting class with the Orlando Shakespeare Theater, (OST). I was going to miss the first class, but the staff approved my admission. When I made it to the second workshop, the other class members were surprised I had only been in Orlando four days. Later, the managing director invited me to participate in a workshop for original show, *St. Joan*.

At the Osceola Performing Arts Center I received the *Best Performance from a Newcomer* for my performance of Arry in *Morning's at Seven*. The irony was that the playwright, Paul Osborne, was from Kalamazoo and the characters were based on his aunts who lived next door to each other. There was a stipulation that the play could not be performed in Kalamazoo as long as the aunts were alive. To the best of my knowledge, the play has only been produced twice in town.

One of the ladies in the Royal National Theatre group had given me the name of an agent in Orlando. I made an appointment and at our first meeting I was signed on and sent on several commercial auditions. I was so excited the first time I went to Universal Studios. To be where classic movies were made was overwhelming for this small-town girl. I walked up to the guard house, gave my name and the uniformed security officer checked me off the list. On the way to the sound stage I made up a little song, "I'm on the list. Look at me. I'm on the list."

For one audition, I had to hula-hoop, and another I dressed up like a nun. But the most memorable audition was when I flew to Miami for a Denzel Washington movie, *Out of Time*. He wasn't there, of course. I didn't get the role and none of the auditions garnered any employment. I believe if I had stayed longer, I would have had more opportunities of securing a commercial or two. Right before I left, I was offered a job at the Orlando Shakespeare Festival. It was an offer I couldn't, but had to refuse.

2001 - After the worst day in US history, September 11, Rich was riffed (reduction in force), from American Airlines. Nothing could soothe our disappointment and frustration. In hindsight, it was a blessing in disguise. Rich had been working sixty hours a week and the stress was taking its toll. I was worried about him and his health because he had lost a lot of weight.

In the past we had always lived in condos or apartments. Four months before being riffed, we had purchased our very first house. We were settled in and had made it our own. With the new development, we didn't know where we were going or what we were going to do.

Ultimately rescued by a friend, Rich was offered a job in Gainesville, FL with Delta Airlines. When he went off to start his new job, I stayed in Orlando to take care of selling the house. When the movers came and the house was completely empty, I sat in the middle of the living room and sobbed.

To the citizens of Gainesville, FL, you have a lovely town. I tried the local theatre scene and would have been cast in *Moon Over Buffalo*. Fortunately, or unfortunately, we had a much-needed vacation planned and I was going to miss a large portion of rehearsal time.

I worked as the Box Office Manager at the Hippodrome and enjoyed it. But I just didn't fit in there and I was miserable. We almost purchased a house, but something in my head told me not to go through with it.

2002 - It was a happy day in June when Susan called to tell us that by December we were going to be grandparents. I was excited, but upset because I didn't want to be a long-distance grandma. I begged Rich to do whatever he could do to find a job in Kalamazoo. I knew a job wasn't going to fall out of the sky, but we had to find a way to get back home.

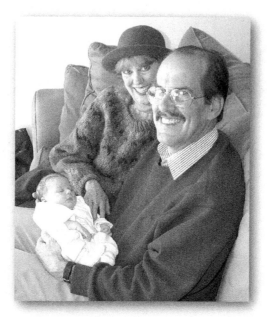

2002 Hannah's proud grandparents.

As I re-read my memoir I've noticed that with every disastrous situation we've been pulled out in the nick of time. "When God closes a door, he opens a window?" Someone, or something continues to watch over our lives.

One of Rich's air traffic control friends was working for a privately-owned ATC company and was getting ready to retire. He highly recommended Rich, and because Rich knew others working there, he was hired. We moved again. And I was home for the birth of our granddaughter, Hannah, On December 30, 2002.

2005 - In 2005 The Kalamazoo Promise was initiated. Kalamazoo high school students who maintain their grades receive tuition free college. I've included this because I am so proud of my community. There are so many opportunities for young people to succeed. Other cities are adopting a plan fashioned after The Promise[+8]

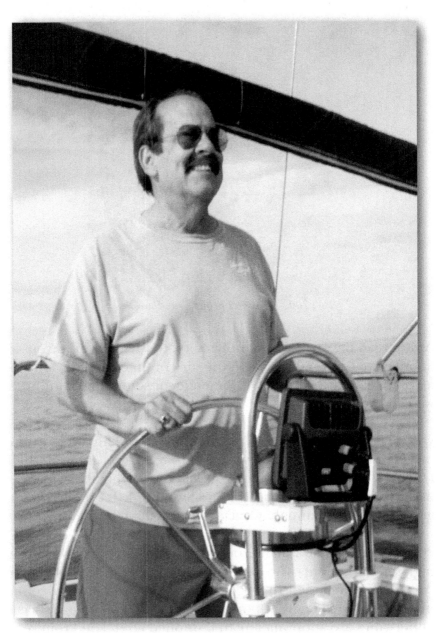

Anna Maria Island 2016. Rich's first sailing adventure.

Chapter 5
A LONG DAY'S JOURNEY INTO NIGHT

By 2003 a long-time friend, Duwain Hunt, held the Managing Director position for the Kalamazoo Civic Theatre. When he learned I was back in town, he offered me a job as the National Host Chair for the 2005 American Association of Community Theaters Festival or *AACTFest* for short. I gladly accepted, and was happy to be back working in my beloved theatre.

Michigan Governor Jennifer Granholm had named Kalamazoo a "*Cool City*," so I coined the festival: "*A Hot Time in The Cool City*." Twenty-six theatres, five hundred people from all over the country, plus one from Germany, converged on Kalamazoo to present their best plays or musicals. The week was filled with theatre competitions, adjudications, and awards. My job was to register all theatres and participants, arrange for hotel rooms, and design two brochures plus the main program. Our technical staff made sure the participants had everything they needed in the way of additional props or set pieces. They also helped them set proper levels for their own lighting and sound designs. All of the performances were adjudicated by three reputable leaders in community theatre. The winners were given awards, bragging rights and were often invited to international festivals. In 1997, James Carver's production of *Dancing at Lughnasa* took first place in the state and regional competitions. The company was invited to perform in the highly esteemed international festival in Monaco. Rich and I tagged along to cheer them on.

During the Kalamazoo festival, I realized my breathing was getting worse. And yet, like an idiot, I continued to smoke. With *AACTFest* completed, I made an appointment with a pulmonologist to acquire a smoking cessation drug.

There were so many doctors for so many reasons over the next few years, so without naming names, I'll use an alphabetical list. The first session with Dr. "A" did not go well. His bedside manner was nonexistent. Flippantly he told me, "Find something else to do with your hands." When I responded with, "I tried that but almost got arrested," he didn't appreciate my sense of humor.

After examining me, he said the words I never wanted to hear, "You have emphysema." I think I had an outer body experience because I don't remember anything else after that. My thoughts immediately rushed back to my father and how he suffered. He didn't have an oxygen tank, so after a few steps he would collapse, wherever he was, and gasp for breath. It was frightening and sad at the same time. To see this vibrant man, the man who loved to fish and hunt and swim, struggling to breathe. And now I was facing that same future.

It wasn't the diagnosis that inspired me to find another doctor. I tried working with him for two more appointments but decided we were not a good match. I knew that if I was going to be faced with this devastating illness, I needed a doctor who had a little more compassion. I started looking for another pulmonologist. I felt empowered when I sashayed into Dr. "A"'s office and demanded my medical records. They knew I would not be back. Later, when I started physical therapy, I learned other patients did not care for his attitude. I asked why they kept going back but they didn't have an answer.

Actually, that first experience wasn't all bad. Dr. "A" prescribed much needed oxygen. I knew I needed it, but I panicked the day the huge tanks, refillable portables and concentrator were delivered. [+9]I was only fifty-six years old. I was too young for this. I knew nothing about oxygen—only that it could explode. I worried that our home and lives could go up in smoke. I presumed I would have to be attached to this contraption for the rest of my life and there was a question as to how long that life would be. But I had to deal with it. I had to learn how to use the hideous beast; what settings were beneficial, when to raise or lower the Liters Per Minute (LPM) and how long the tubing needed to be for maximum usage. And then there's the cannula—two prongs sticking up my nostrils. This did not make an impressive fashion statement. The line from *Welcome Back Kotter* came to mind, "Up your nose with a rubber hose." To avoid that image, I started referring to it as my nose jewelry. But my horrible confession is this: I was so addicted to cigarettes, I would take the cannula out of my nose, turn off the oxygen, and go outside on our deck for a cigarette. DUMB.

Susan
"Before surgery, seeing my mom on oxygen. Sad . . . Seeing my mom take off her oxygen and head out to the deck for a smoke. Mad . . . I understand how hard it is to stop smoking – it has taken me years to do so – but URGH."

Another little gadget I became acquainted with was the pulse oximeter or *pulse ox* for short. Now if you've ever been hospitalized, your nurse or technician has taken your vitals—more often than not, waking you from a sound sleep. They measure blood pressure, temperature, and they use the pulse ox to measure your pulse and oxygen levels. Many people with Chronic Obstructive Pulmonary Disease (COPD) or other lung diseases own a meter and have it by their side at all times. With 100% being the highest level, my reading was 25% at the time of my diagnosis. With so little oxygen, it was extremely difficult to walk. It felt like I weighed a thousand pounds. To move even two feet was exhausting.

It amazes me how adaptable humans are in adverse situations. After a few months of living with oxygen, it became as natural as chewing gum. I dubbed my portable "Wheezy," and she went with me everywhere. If I was going to do anything strenuous I would proclaim, "Turn up the juice and turn me loose." I would put her on the side of the pool to continue with my low-impact water-aerobics class appropriately named *Jaws and Joints* because we worked both.

There were drawbacks, sure. We lived in a three-story condo. For access to all areas, I needed fifty feet of tubing which was a neon shade of green. I certainly couldn't hide from anyone. Just follow the snake and I would be at the end. Visitors had to learn how to jump rope, but I never made them do Double Dutch. When I was giving Rich some grief, he thought it was funny to bend the tubing—giving a whole new meaning to the word kinky. And when the green snake got wrapped around my leg, I performed moves the Rockettes would envy.

The tubing also created a problem while rising from a chair, or unfortunately the toilet. I would step on the tube and it would yank my head down. Or the cannula would jerk out of my nose. Countless times a day I would get caught on something: doors, drawer pulls, chairs, the dishwasher, the dog. When I carried any liquid from the kitchen to the living room I would often trip. The beverage would jump out of the cup splattering all over the floor, while expletives shot out of my mouth. For atonement, I thanked God for hardwood floors.

The condo we purchased in 2002 had wall to wall carpeting in every room, except kitchen and bath. After one incontinent dog, several parties, and many, many spills later, it was not in great shape. Taking my health into consideration, we purchased hardwood floors throughout. The air was cleaner, and it gave my lungs a healthy environment. My sister Rosemary offered her home during the installation so my lungs weren't compromised from the dust.

Dr. "A" also wrote a prescription for pulmonary rehab classes that were extremely beneficial. The large exercise room consisted of rowing bikes, treadmills, weights, resistance bands, medicine balls, pulls, and a barre. One of the members dubbed this class *The Heavy Breathers*. We started with fifteen wonderful people, all older than me, at different stages of lung disease. When the facility closed after a year, we met for lunch on the third Thursday of every month. At the end of every luncheon, although unspoken, we wondered how many would be around the following month. Several lunches and funerals later, the numbers dwindled, and by 2015 everyone had passed except me. Because of their age, they didn't have the option of transplantation.

There was a wonderful day when I had a "teachable moment." Rich and I were in a restaurant while sitting kitty corner from us were two young boys . . . both parents were on their cell phones. Don't get me started on that one. That's another book. The little boy, about eight or nine years old, was staring. I smiled and waved, and this continued throughout our meal. On our way out, I stopped by their table.

Me:	Hi, what's your name?
Little Boy:	Tommy.
Me:	Well Tommy, it seems like you were curious about this. (*I pointed to the cannula and the oxygen. He shook his head yes. His brother was not at all interested.*)
Me:	I have trouble breathing so this device supplies me with oxygen so I can move easily. I call her Wheezy.
Tommy:	That's cool.
Me:	Would you like to hear it? (*He nodded his head yes again. I took the cannula out of my nose, turned the oxygen up to continuous flow so he could feel the cool breeze. I then held it up to his ear*).
Tommy:	Oh, WOW.

Me: Now when you see someone with this or a similar
             device, you'll know what it's for.
Tommy: Thanks.

His parents thanked me profusely and we all smiled and said goodbye. My inner devil wanted to say, "Put down your freakin' phones
and pay attention to your kids." But my inner angel made me be
nice. I can only imagine the next day at school, he would tell the
story of the lady with the tube in her nose and how he got to listen
to it. He would be the hero of the day, and quite frankly, I felt like
a hero as well.

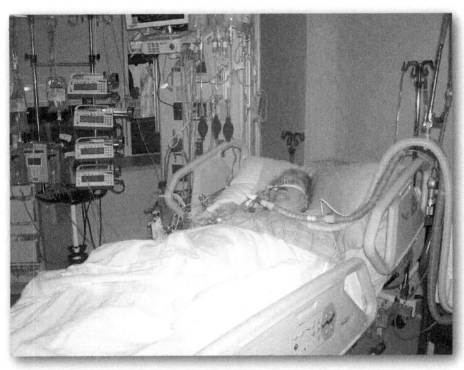

2008 – University of Michigan Hospital. Lifesaving machines.

Chapter 6
DEATH TRAP

In 2006, a friend recommended another physician, Dr. "B," so I made an appointment with him. The first time we met we got along famously. He prescribed a cigarette-cessation medication and for legality's sake, let's call it "Smoke Not." The side effects included, agitation, dry mouth, constipation, headache/migraine, nausea/ vomiting, excessive sweating, dizziness, tremors, and drowsiness. On the way home, around noon, I had the prescription filled, took one tablet, and slept for most of the day. I awoke in a fog, made dinner, watched some TV and at 9 p.m. I was ready to go to bed, so I took another pill.

Minutes after taking the capsule, I was doubled over in pain and I couldn't catch my breath. I was downstairs, Rich was upstairs on the computer in the same room as the concentrator. With all the strength I could muster, I "yelled" for him to turn the LPM as high as it would go. When nothing happened, I knew something was horribly wrong. Our Cairn Terrier, Kyna, (pronounced Kī - nuh) knew it, too. She was whimpering, pacing back and forth. When I crawled my way to our miniscule half-bath, she was right by my side.

Gasping for breath, this time I screamed, "CALL 911." The para-medics arrived in ten minutes and tried to unbend me, but it was excruciating. They administered more oxygen and started an IV.

If it hadn't been so petrifying, it might have been comical. There was a big burly guy and a big burly gal, my dog, and me, all in this teeny tiny bathroom. Rich was outside the door looking in. He wanted Kyna to get out, but I wanted her in, "Leave her alone," I yelled. "She's scared." The EMTs were trying to do their best under difficult circumstances.

The last thing I remember was being outside in the cold, lying on the gurney, and being shoved into the ambulance. At the end of our driveway I lost consciousness. To this day I swear I do not remember anything that happened after that.

Rich explained that when we arrived at Bronson's emergency room I was in so much pain I was letting everyone know it by using all the raunchy words not listed in Webster's Dictionary. It is alleged that I said, "Stop that, you son of a b****. Quit it, you a** hole. Mother f****," and on and on. I don't know how he kept a straight face when he innocently told them, "She never talks like that."

When I finally opened my eyes, it was surreal. Staring at the grey ceiling, amid the repugnant hospital smells, I was intubated, (*a tube was inserted into my trachea for ventilation.*) My wrists and ankles were in restraints. I thought of the 1948 movie, *The Snake Pit*, where Olivia de Havilland wakes up and finds herself in an insane asylum and can't remember how she got there. I didn't realize how much time had passed and was shocked to learn it was the following morning . . . twelve hours later. I was so thankful to see Susan sitting in the recliner. Rich had just left to purchase breakfast for them.

When Doctor "C" entered the room, he told us I was a very lucky lady. If we had waited ten minutes more to call 911, I would have been dead. Reality check. I thought back to a childhood neighbor who nicknamed me "Cat Eyes." Well, if I am a cat, I'd just lost one of my nine lives.

A good friend of ours was a Physician Assistant (P.A.). He heard about the incident and visited me in the ICU the day after it happened. When he walked in, I was sitting up in bed, chatting and laughing with Rich, Susan and one of the nurses. He stopped in his tracks.

PA   "I thought you'd be . . ."
Me   (I finished it for him.) "Dead?"
PA   (While stammering) "Yes . . . well, no, but I didn't think you would be holding court."

After the emergency had passed and everyone left the room, Doctor "C" came back to discuss my situation. "I know what happened," I said. "I took Smoke Not and ended up in the emergency room." He shook his head in disagreement. I argued, "It was the only thing I did differently in my medication routine and I hadn't eaten anything unusual." He continued to disagree and I perceived his attitude as, "What do you know, you're not a doctor." I don't think he ever had a patient who challenged him. I could tell he didn't like it and, after a few minutes, he finally left the room. I wondered why he wouldn't even consider my idea. I have my theories, but I'll let you draw your own conclusions.

I looked up "Smoke Not" on the internet and sent an email to the Company's CEO. They needed to know how this drug affected me and in the long run prevent others from having a similar experience. Two weeks later, I received the typical form letter-sorry for your experience, blah, blah, blah. We need a doctor's signature before any action can be taken, blah, blah, blah. So, I dropped it knowing the doctor wouldn't sign anything. I silently prayed it wouldn't happen to anyone else.

Even though I liked Dr. "B," my trust in him was shattered by the December 6th episode so I was apprehensive about returning to him.

I contacted Dr. "D" and was assigned a Physician's Assistant. This woman was awesome. She spent forty-five minutes with me on the first visit, answered all of my questions, and was genuinely interested in my case. My lung function continued to deteriorate and after several appointments and with much anxiety, I asked her if I had any options, other than to make sure my will was in order. She educated me on double lung transplants and referred me for an appointment at the University of Michigan (U of M) Hospital in Ann Arbor.

Even though I was given all the risks and life expectancy, I never hesitated in proceeding with the idea. I was amazed that anything like that existed and thought wouldn't it have been wonderful if my dad had had the same opportunity.

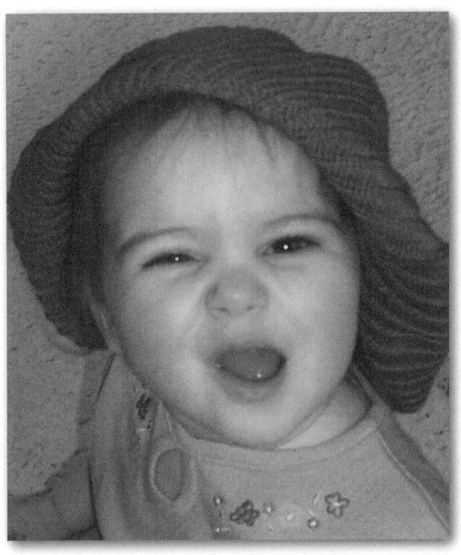

Granddaughter Hannah showing her personality.

Chapter 7
DOUBT

The first time we went to U of M, we asked our P.A. friend to go with us. Luckily, he agreed. Even though transplants were not his area of expertise, we were confident he could interpret the medical jargon. The three of us were escorted into a drab waiting room complete with art work reminiscent of Walmart's finest. I thought if brighter colors would be used in hospitals it might benefit patients' attitudes.

When Dr. "E" entered the room, there was an immediate bond. Because he has been with me through the entire process he deserves more than a letter! Dr. Kevin Chan was/and is charming, caring, informative. He spent over an hour with us covering the determining factors for lung transplantation and answered all the questions we knew to ask. Since the December 6th episode, I had forsworn cigarettes. He validated that a candidate had to be smoke free for an entire year before being considered for the surgery.

Another criterion for becoming a transplant candidate was to complete a list of medical procedures to determine my general health. When I had completed a specific procedure, the qualifying doctor would sign and date the list. If the procedures were not completed in a year's time, I would have to start from the beginning. Tests included heart catheterization, echocardiogram, mammogram, pap smear, colonoscopy, bronchoscopy, blood work, bone density, and Hepatitis C. I was picked, patted, poked, probed, pinned, and punctured.

When I went for my Hepatitis C test, Dr. "F" conveyed the results had returned as positive. I was speechless but that didn't last long. "YOU ARE CLEARLY MISTAKEN," I countered. I was familiar with the causes after reading information on line. I hadn't indulged in any sexual misconduct, nor had I used any dirty needles. I hadn't swapped bodily fluids with anyone other than my hubby, but Dr. "F" was adamant. I argued that if she reported these bogus results, it would bring my check-list to a screeching halt. I only had a limited amount of time to finish testing. When she refused to back down, I knew I had get a second opinion. I found Doctor "G" and the same day the results came back negative. Situations like this taught me to trust my knowledge, my intuition and to ask questions when I felt something was incorrect.

The first of many lung function tests was conducted by an African American man, (wait for the punch line), who was all business. So serious. He guided me to an area consisting of his very small desk, a computer, and a spaceship-like chamber. I was handed a plastic clothespin-like device to put on my nose, the purpose being not to let air escape. I was also handed an apparatus that stretched out my mouth. A dentist once told me, "No one can ever say you have a big mouth." Well, some people might disagree with that.

The chamber door closed with the sound of grinding gears. I'd love to know how they dealt with claustrophobic patients 'cause it's TIGHT in there. I resisted the impulse to say, "Beam me up, Scotty." The technician spoke through a microphone with speakers inside the chamber. It was similar to a God mike in the theatre and his voice sounded like it came from above. He directed me to follow a sing-songy breathing pattern and demonstrated by whistling. "Now follow what I do," he said. I tried and tried, but every time I mangled the entire phrase. I could tell his frustration was building. To ease the tension I finally declared, "You know white girls don't have no rhythm." His stoic demeanor rapidly changed and he burst into gales of laughter. We had fun with it after that.

Another requirement before being placed on the organ transplant list was a mandatory meeting for family members and caregivers. Rich, Susan, Susan's husband, Rosemary and I all attended. There were five other candidates facing the same circumstances. We were re-introduced to our transplant team, Dr. Chan and Ros, who became not only my lung transplant coordinator, but my confidant. We also met a social worker and Dr. "H," the surgeon who would be performing the operation. Each staff member described their jobs. They verified what we could expect from them and provided us with details about what to anticipate before, during and after the operation.

We were given the opportunity to ask any questions, however some of the answers were disturbing: "This will not be a cure for your problems. In fact, you will be trading one set of problems for another. There is no guarantee that the transplant will work. Life after this point will be challenging and taxing. It takes a dedicated support team to help you through it. The recipient will be in a great deal of pain after the operation. They will be taking narcotics such as OxyContin, Vicodin, etc. so they need someone to manage and regulate their medication."

Luckily, I had a fabulous support team with Rich, Susan, and Rosemary. As we drove back to Kalamazoo, we had much to think about and discuss.

Susan
At U of M, my mom, my dad, and I listening to a lung transplant consultation before being put on the waiting list. This was a very scary meeting. Everything was going to change in my family's lives, whether she got a pair of lungs or didn't. The one point I remember the most is it is very rare for a patient to live longer than 10 years after the surgery. The life expectancy odds mentioned in the pamphlet kept depleting each year.

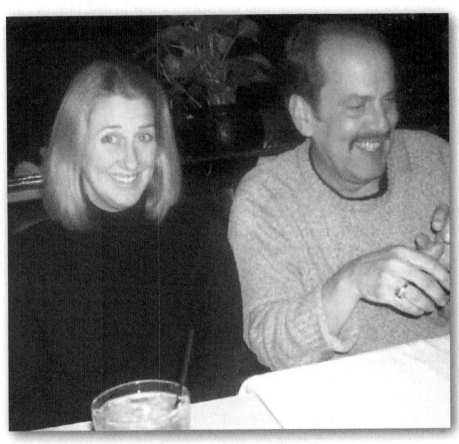

January 21, 2008. Transplant surgery. No better time for a drink.

Chapter 8
THE MIRACLE WORKER

By the time I finished all the testing, it was October 2007. I must have been high priority because after being placed on the list, I only waited three months to get the call. I've read that some candidates wait as long as three years. Many don't live long enough for donor organs to become available.

I screamed into the phone when the good news came on a Sunday. Rich was doing the grocery shopping, so I called his cell phone,

"Are you almost done?" I'm surprised he didn't hear the excitement in my voice because he sounded annoyed,

"What'd you forget?"

"Oh, I didn't forget anything, but they do have a set of lungs waiting for me at the hospital."

"I'LL BE RIGHT HOME." he yelled.

And yes, he did manage to pay for the groceries before hightailing it home.

Susan had made arrangements for Family Emergency Leave, so I hung up and called her immediately. She was at our house in fifteen minutes and we started our drive.

From the very beginning, we were told that once we received the call, we had four hours to make it to the hospital otherwise another recipient would receive the lungs. It takes two hours to get to Ann Arbor from Kalamazoo. Rich confessed he did not stay within the speed limit. That was obvious because we were there in an hour and forty-five minutes.

> *Susan*
> *Getting the call: lungs are in. It seemed fast – we didn't wait long for the donation (3 months?) Grabbing all my stuff to go with my parents to Ann Arbor. Making sure my five-year-old daughter was going to be taken care of. Driving in scared silence – I don't remember talking too much on the way there. We got there and then: Waiting, waiting, waiting, and mom was finally admitted, waiting, waiting, deciding to get food and drinks, exhausted, waiting, going back to the hospital, sleeping or barely sleeping in the chairs while waiting. Finally seeing the doctor who performed the transplant – he looked like he was hit by a truck. He said something about taking her off the bypass was tricky and the whole procedure took eight hours. We would eventually be able to see her but we have to wait. Yup, waited some more.*

It amazes me how calm we were considering where we were headed and what we were facing. We were known as "the fun family," but this was a critical moment. As the miles ticked by, I couldn't help but think of the donor's family. We were on our way to the unknown . . . an optimistic beginning. While another family, in another hospital, was facing finality. Saying goodbye to their loved one for the very last time must have been heartbreaking.

I knew that Jean, one of my Heavy Breather friends, wanted to know when I received the much-awaited news. We shared a fascination with the supernatural and she loved guessing people's astrological signs. Shortly after we met she had a dream that we were together as kids, holding hands and skipping on a dock in

Saugatuck. Uncanny. Another remarkable fact, her husband, John, was from Chicago and lived three blocks from the Weirs. He went to the same high school as Rich. Years before, of course, but even so . . .

I called to tell her the good news. There was a rule in her house that on Sundays, whenever the Chicago Bears were playing, no calls were allowed. She was a huge fan and so was Rich. When the phone rang that day, she was irritated. Continuing with her glass of wine she told her daughter, Randi, to answer it. Randi relays what happened next, "*When my mom found out it was Cathie, I swear I never saw her move so fast in my life. She nearly killed herself tripping over the ottoman to get to the phone.*"

Knowing that the future was questionable, we had a heart to heart talk, but managed to squeeze in a few laughs. Jean wished me well and we said goodbye. Shortly after the operation, she admitted that she didn't think I was going to make it. Unfortunately, she passed away on February 28, 2015.

I have been asked if I felt guilty about receiving someone's lungs. I'm not sure if that's a valid question. I felt empathy for the family, I felt compassion and grateful that this option was available, but how could I feel guilty about something over which I had no control? The purpose of organ donation is so others may live. To my good fortune, my donor family made that decision. As of this writing, I have not met my donor family, but whoever they are, I will always be indebted to them.

When we arrived at the hospital I was prepped with an I.V. and my vitals were taken. I was going to be given massive doses of Prednisone which makes the body swell. I couldn't remove my precious jewelry, grandmother's and mother's wedding bands so they had to be cut off. That was distressing, but luckily, I was able to slide my own wedding band and engagement ring off my finger. They were saved.

When we read the legal papers to sign, my situation became frighteningly clear. There was the Advanced Directive: *A written statement of a person's wishes regarding medical treatment, often including a living will, made to ensure those wishes are carried out should the person be unable to communicate them to a doctor.* Wills had been drawn for both of us by my brother-in-law Alan Burke. We had taken care of that in the months prior.

The one paper that alarmed the three of us was the DNR: *Do Not Resuscitate is a legal order written either in the hospital or on a legal form to withhold cardiopulmonary resuscitation (CPR) or advanced cardiac life support (ACLS), in respect of the wishes of a patient should he or she were to stop breathing.* It was alarming to face the fact that something could go wrong and this could be the end of my life. I'm not often shaken, but under those circumstances, I buckled. With Rich and Susan expressing words of encouragement, I rallied and signed it with an affirmative. I don't believe in extending life if there is no quality of life. I didn't want my family to be saddled with any unwanted burdens. They had been through enough up to this point.

We waited and waited and ultimately learned the organs hadn't been harvested yet. I believe it was five hours before they finally took me to the operating room. Rich and Susan headed to the bar for much needed cocktails. I would have gone as well had I been coherent enough. Even though the air was filled with anxiety, instead of saying goodbye, we said, **"I'll see you later."**

In the operating room, I met the surgeon, Dr. "H" for the second time. "Are you ready?" he said. "Are you?" I countered. "How much coffee have you had? I'm a little nervous about you shaking in the middle of cutting me open." He laughed, but then quickly asked for the anesthesiologist to knock me out.

Taking a long razor-sharp scalpel, they sliced me starting under my left breast to my right. I'd always been chesty, but by now my coconuts had fallen far from the tree. I wondered what they did with my boobs so they didn't get in the way. Afterwards, I told Jean they duct taped them to my shoulders. Her eyes became as big as saucers and it took her a second before she realized I was joking.

My ribs were broken to have access to the lungs. If you've ever had a broken bone, you know the pain. They took the Jaws of Life (kidding) and squeezed my ribs back so the doctors could jump in and do their deed. While I was hooked up to the bypass machine, they carefully removed one bad lung and replaced it with the new one. Once they determined the new lung was functioning correctly, they replaced the other one. Then a steel rod was placed to provide something solid for the ribs to be attached. I was stapled up with the "clam shell" technique.

When I groggily woke up from the eight-hour surgery, my wrists and ankles were in restraints again. I had IV's in both arms, a central line in my neck, and chest tubes draining fluid from my laceration. I was intubated, and a piece of rod was sticking out of my chest.

To ease the intense pain, I was given a morphine drip button, but I could only push it every seven minutes. I watched the clock like a hawk and at the appropriate time, I'd thrust the plunger down with glee sending a nice buzz through my veins. I loved the morphine . . . almost too much. And I loved the automatic leg compression socks which pulsated every two minutes. It was a fabulous leg massage.

Using American Sign Language, (which I learned while performing in *Children of a Lesser God*), I motioned to Susan, WTF. And get this hose out of my throat. And I want a drink of water, my throat is sore. Pleasantly, she said, "Not until the nurse comes in." When the nurse came in, she made me promise not to yank on the tube.

I nodded in agreement, and it came out slowly and agonizingly. My throat felt like sandpaper for the next week.

> *Susan*
> *Mom waking up from the surgery. She still had tubes down her throat. She was having a hard time with them. She started moving her hands, she was doing something with her hands that are tied down . . . signing with her hands . . . W . . . A . . . T . . . E . . . WATER, no I'm sorry mom you can't have water until they take the tubes out. Nurses in and out . . . NOT TAKING THE TUBES OUT... What the . . . come on . . . take the tubes out . . . take the tubes out . . . she's in pain.*

During the two-week stay, Susan kept a log showing how many people came in and out of my room in the days following my surgery. The list is dated January 29, 2008, but it reflects how many interruptions there were per day. On this particular day, there were close to forty "visits," but some days there were more.

Susan	*1/29/08*
8:40	*Nurse Michelle*
8:45	*Blood Draw*
8:47	*Cleaning supplies*
8:50	*Daily Menu*
8:51	*Nurse Michelle – Tylenol*
9:06	*Nurse Michelle – Meds*
9:07	*Dr. Alsuiee – Cardiology*
9:29	*Clean linen – Tech guy, Ted*
9:47	*Dr. Yen – Transplant Team*
10:00	*Dr. Yen*
10:01	*Nurse Michelle – Meds*
10:10	*Nurse Michelle – enema*
10:41	*Dr. Morris*
10:42	*Gatorade delivery*
10:47	*Echo heart*
10:53	*Nurse Michelle – oxygen tanks*

10:56	*Respiratory – three people*
11:15	*Dr. Candelle – PA*
11:16	*Nurse Michelle*
11:20	*Walk*
11:30	*RN Walls – post transplant team*
11:49	*Nurse Michelle*
11:51	*RN Walls and Ros – transplant coordinators*
11:56	*Tech – Ted – Blood sugar – 104*
12:22	*Lunch*
12:52	*Dr. Candela – Thorasic*
1:03	*Newspaper delivery*
1:13	*Nurse Michelle – noon meds*
1:37	*Pick up lunch tray*
2:00	*Michelle – meds*
2:17	*Physical therapy*
2:17	*Blood draw*
2:22	*Laura – diabetes discussion*
2:30	*Nurse Michelle*
2:57	*Transplant team – five people*

One of my biggest complaints was that no one ever remembered to close the door. I didn't want to hear any noise, especially other people screaming in pain, and I didn't want to hear the incessant chatter from the staff. The room I had after surgery was right across the hall from the nurse's station. Remember in the past there were signs that said QUIET – HOSPITAL ZONE? Well, that didn't apply here. I wanted to sleep, but there was to be no sleeping in this hospital. They woke me up in the middle of the night to tell me I had to go to the bathroom or check my vitals. I <u>did</u> <u>not</u> have to go to the bathroom, either number one or number two. I was sleeping and I was hooked up to numerous machines monitoring my every move, so why in the heck did they have to wake me up at all?

After the catheter was taken out, going to the bathroom meant a bed-pan or, my preference, the commode. This little porta potty was quite convenient. All I had to do was stand up and swing my butt around and do my business in the "hat." What a ridiculous name for a human waste collector. The nurses would then take the "hat," and measure the contents. I'm telling you, those nurses are saints.

More and more staff members wanted to talk to me, but they all asked the same questions, "How are you feeling? On a scale of one to ten, how is your pain? Any vomiting or diarrhea? After the eighty-ninth time, I finally said, "Don't you people talk to each other? And even if you don't it's all listed in the computer." One doctor's reply was rather clever. He said, "We want to hear it from you." Well, I DIDN'T WANT TO TALK. My throat was raw from the tubing, I was barely coherent, my ribcage was killing me, and I had painful IV's. Who wants to talk under those circumstances?" Rich was very polite with the doctors and explained how frustrating it was for me to communicate, especially when the process was so redundant. I finally signed a paper that authorized Rich to speak for me. After that, whenever anyone came in the room, I just pointed to him. He became my voice . . . just another reason why I appreciate him so much.

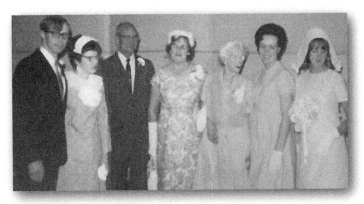

1969 – The last time the entire family was together.

Chapter 9
HOMECOMING

After two brutal weeks, which seemed like two months, I was released from the hospital along with a grocery bag filled with medication. We have a marble topped buffet, eight feet by two feet, and when all our treasured tchotchkes were removed, the drugs filled the entire surface. They included anti-rejection, anti-viral, antibiotics, anti-fungal, stool softeners, anti-nausea, vitamins, a nebulizer, insulin, blood thinner, enema paraphernalia, and a spirometer, [+10] which I nicknamed suck and blow.

One of the most frustrating elements of recovery was regression. For every two steps forward, I would take ten steps back. I would resolve one issue and feel fabulous, but then another would pop up. It was so frustrating and disheartening. I thought I was never going to feel well again. It was always due to the medications. The doctors continually searched for the right cocktail to make me healthier, but we're not talkin' rum and coke here.

> You know the song *Go Ask Alice?*
> In my case, it was:
> One pill made me vomit.
> One pill made me poop.
> And the one the doctors gave me,
> Just sent me for a loop.

Seriously, one pill made me so high all I wanted to do was sit around and listen to *In-A-Gadda-Da-Vida* at full blast . . . with the base turned up. With the doctor's permission, I stopped taking that drug. I couldn't concentrate and I had no control over anything. I now understand why people get hooked on medications. When you're hurting, (mentally and physically), you'll do anything to alleviate the pain. I was around heavy drugs in the 70's and 80's; cocaine, LSD, but I never had any desire to partake. Just a little grass made me happy.

Rosemary and Alan, were living in Indiana at the time of my release. She generously offered to stay with me for a couple of weeks while Rich was at work. Rosemary earned her RN in 1960 but hadn't practiced in a long time. Rosemary was/is the brains of the family. She graduated from Nazareth with a Bachelor of Business Administration, Summa Cum Laude in 1984. Went on to graduate from the University of Notre Dame with a Master of Science in Administration in 1987, In 1992 she graduated from ND Law School. Needless to say, I felt safe with her overseeing this complicated process.

There was much to be done: making my meals, managing my drugs, changing the soiled bandages under my boobs every day. Because of my tender Prednisone skin, the removal of bandages was often more painful than the wound itself. Rosemary had to empty drainage tubes and measure their contents.

While in the hospital, I was shattered to learn I had Prednisone induced diabetes. I thought, Good God, what else are you going to throw at me? So, I had to learn how to give myself shots of insulin two or three times a day, but if I wasn't feeling well, Rosemary would take over the task. A blood thinner, Lovanox, we called it Love Nuts, required another piercing, so my fingers and stomach were a delightful rainbow of colors: black, blue, green and purple.

Besides friends, an army of visiting home nurses, physical thera-pists who helped me with exercises to build up my strength, and counselors were in and out the door. Whenever anyone visited, Rosemary channeled Nurse Ratchet from *One Flew Over the Cuckoo's Nest*. Guests had to immerse themselves in Purell and wear protec-tive masks. They were allotted fifteen minutes, no more, no less. When the time was up, my sister would scream, "**OUT**." And out they went. Rosemary also "encouraged," aka nagged, me to get up and walk around the condo. "It's good for the bowels" she'd say. I just wanted to curl up in my comfy, cozy, snug as a bug bed and go to sleep.

It was wonderful to be home but very challenging. I needed help getting in and out of the bath tub/shower, so we purchased a shower chair. I couldn't get up from the toilet . . . that was embarrassing, and my legs and feet had to be lifted into the bed. I couldn't drive for four months because I was filled with narcotics and I couldn't lift more than ten pounds. For a Type A personality, all of these limitations were problematic.

Our beautiful Carin Terrier, Kyna, had to be shipped out because no fur friends were allowed. My lovely niece Katie, Rosemary's daughter, offered to take her in. Katie also had experience deal-ing with indisposed patients. With that and cleaning my house and doing laundry every Tuesday, she was a godsend.

Not being able to see my granddaughter was another disadvan-tage. We spoke on the phone, but as we all know, kids carry germs, and germs were verboten. In the first few weeks back home, every little sniff, sneeze, cough or spit had to be recorded. Any germ could send me right back into the hospital.

Along with surgery there came a certain amount of blood and gore. At first, I was frightened when I coughed into the pink plastic bin and saw droplets of blood. Then, of course, there was bleeding from my wound. To cover my angst, I did my best impression of Rosanne Rosannadanna with, "Did that come out of me?" It was calming when my transplant coordinator, Ros, told me not to worry unless the blood secretions were more than a Tablespoon.

We have a three-story home: basement, main floor, bedrooms upstairs. There are seven stairs going up or down, a landing, and seven more steps. The first few nights home from surgery I stayed downstairs on the couch or in the recliner, so I didn't disturb Rich's sleep.

Susan came up with the idea of putting a bench on the landing so I could sleep in the guest bedroom. She surmised it would be more comfortable sleeping there rather than the couch or recliner. She and Rich would help me up the first few steps, let me rest, and then we continued. It was a lot easier going down because I could scoot on my butt.

Physical therapy played an important role for my recovery. In ICU, they had me up and walking around the day after the surgery. There was so much pain. The nurses wrapped a safety belt around my waist to have control if I were to fall. Two nurses, on either side held me up and another nurse held on to the rolling pole carrying the IV lines. They always had encouraging words like, "you can do this" or "great job." I said thanks, but it was killing me. I liked it better when Rich and Susan were there to help. They would try to make me laugh, but then that hurt as well. I gradually improved to walking slowly up and down the make shift stairs, one at a time.

Susan had a treadmill in her garage that was collecting dust so she found some young men to bring it to our home. I felt sorry for them because it was HEAVY. I was excited when I did ONE minute, a couple of days later THREE minutes, then SEVEN minutes . . . all the way up to THIRTY minutes. The adage "baby steps" was never more accurate.

I was getting back on my feet. There was, however, a yin and yang to my recovery.

- My doctors suggested I shouldn't go swimming. That was like a death sentence to me. Mom said I was swimming before I was walking, so I couldn't stop now.
- My doctors suggested I shouldn't garden because of mold in the dirt. Well, eventually I did do a little gardening, while wearing two masks and two pairs of gloves.
- My doctors suggested I shouldn't have a pet, but my dogs were my fur babies. I took care of them and it made me feel useful. Our first rescue, Kyna, was failing and I knew I couldn't be without a dog. So, we rescued a three-year-old Cairn Terrier I named Kerry. Before she came to live with us, Kyna was acting as though she was on her last legs, but with rambunctious Kerry, she lived for another year, passing away in 2011.

So, I did/and still do all of the above. If I didn't, I wouldn't be living and that's what the transplant was all about.

However, my doctors emphatically insisted that I never stop taking my medication just because I was feeling better. They were full of cautionary tales about patients who stopped taking their meds and ultimately died. I have been vigilant about doing the drugs. But that brings on its own special challenge. You know the commercials for medications that list one hundred and eighty-two side effects and you wonder why anyone would take that particular drug? Here are just a few that transplant survivors often deal with:

- Diverticulitis
- Pulmonary Embolus
- Pneumonia, Anemia
- C-Diff
- E. coli

- Infusions, Transfusions
- Thrush
- High Blood Pressure
- Migraines
- Dry Mouth
- Hair Loss
- Tremors
- Lung Infection
- Kidney Disease
- Gastric Ulcer
- Gastro Paresis
- Hypertension,
- Immunosuppression
- Vitamin D Deficiency
- Diabetes
- Esophago-gastroduodenoscopy (can't even pronounce that one)
- Ileostomy
- Shingles
- Depression

I've had it all. Who wouldn't be depressed after all of that?

After Rosemary left, Rich had to take on her duties while still working as an Air Traffic Controller. I'm amazed that he handled the medical tasks without complaint. He hated watching shows that depicted mangled and bloody body parts and always wanted me to change the channel. I thought it was fascinating. But he was a trooper, cleaning me up after many bouts of diarrhea and vomiting. I'm not sure I would have been as tolerant if the roles had been reversed. I'm extremely lucky he has stayed through all of this. For better, or worse, right? This was the worst.

Recovery wasn't always a bed of roses in the marriage department. There came a point when Rich became a neat freak and we had many arguments about it. I was never a slob, but with so little energy, picking up after myself became a defeating chore. I didn't have the energy to get dressed, let alone run the vacuum cleaner, mop, and become Molly Maid of the Year. I would put something down, let's say a pair of scissors, knowing I was going to use them in a few minutes. I would leave the room, but when I came back they would be gone. Rich had cleaned up after me. We were feeling tension that we'd never felt before. Our roles had been reversed, and it was frustrating.

He took care of me for such a long time, that when I could fend for myself, he had to correct what I was doing. He wanted me to do things his way, put the dishes in the dishwasher, cooking, etc., things I had been doing for forty years. It was frustrating and I couldn't understand why he was behaving that way. Finally, we sat down and I asked him to explain what was happening. He revealed that as an air traffic controller, everything must be precise or people will die. And since my illness, he'd become an expert on dealing with insurance companies where everything must be precise or they won't pay the bills. It became clear after we discussed it. It lightened the mood and restored our relationship. Now when I put something down, I'll yell, "don't touch this," and we break into MC Hammer's *U Can't Touch This*. That's the wonderful thing about having a good marriage. If you're able to sit down and talk things out, you've got a great match.

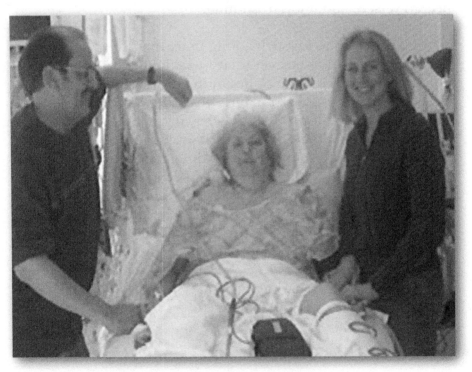

January 21, 2008 – post surgery.

Chapter 10
INHERIT THE WIND

The recipient of any organ is obviously curious about the donor and the donor family. What was the person's age, gender, and how did they pass? How did the donor family make the ultimate decision to go through with the process?

Learning information about the donor family falls under strict parameters. To maintain confidentiality, any correspondence between donor and recipient is conducted through the hospital. The recipient writes a letter to the donor family and delivers it to the hospital staff. The staff then forwards the letter to the donor family and they decide whether or not they want to meet the recipient. I used the University of Michigan's Transplant guidelines to help compose my letter:

- Acknowledge receipt of their gift
- Use your first name only
- Tell about your job or occupation
- Provide a little information about your family (again, first names)
- Tell them about the transplant experience
- Mention how it improved your life
- Don't reveal your address or phone number
- Don't reveal the name of the hospital or physician
- Consider not discussing religion

Just after my transplant, I tried many times to compose a letter that would be empathetic, compassionate, and thankful. But I found it very difficult. How do I express how grateful I was to be alive? How do I convey what their decision has done for me? How could I say I'm travelling—riding horses on the battlefields of Gettysburg, swimming in the Caribbean Sea and listening to a steel band. With all of that and my love of performing and directing again . . . how can I say these things when their loved one has been gone for the same amount of time?

After two years of agonizing over what to say, I went out to the pool with a pen and a legal pad in hand. I sat down and composed this letter:

Dear Donor Family,

I have started this letter over a dozen times but I couldn't find the words to express my deepest gratitude for your gift. My name is Cathie and I am 59 years old. I am the recipient of your loved one's lungs. I was diagnosed with emphysema in 2006. My father died of the disease at age fifty-nine so you can imagine my fear when the doctor broke the news. Because of your generous, unselfish gift, I have lived to celebrate two more birthdays, two more wedding anniversaries, for a total of thirty-nine years, with my husband Rich, birthdays with our daughter, son-in-law, granddaughter, family and many, many friends.

Before the lung transplant I could barely walk 10 steps before stopping to catch my breath. I was on six liters of oxygen and my lung capacity was 25%. Post-surgery my lung capacity has increased to 92%. My husband and I go to the gym three times a week and I participate in a low impact water aerobics class, two days a week. We've always loved to travel but were unable to with my weakened condition. Since the transplant we have visited some of our favorite destinations. My quality of life has increased dramatically.

I can only imagine the grief you must have felt with the loss of your loved one and having to make the heart-wrenching decision to donate their organs. Your loved one lives on in me. I preach the

> *importance of organ donation whenever I get the chance. I hope you have inspired and encouraged others to become donors as well. There are so many others on waiting lists. If you ever decide to meet, I would be more than honored. You are heroes in my eyes. Thank you so much. I owe you my life.*

As of October 2017, I have not met my donor family. In the future, I hope they will want to meet me as much as I want to meet them. By now you know I believe in the supernatural. For whatever reason I believe my lungs are from a young male. I sense a football player, but I could be way off the mark. A nurse slipped one time and said, "You have young lungs. Make sure you take care of them." I shrieked, "Really?" Embarrassed, she replied, "I've said too much."

I've encountered people who give me varying reasons why they won't donate. The most common one, "Nobody would want this ancient body." Please understand that **THERE IS NO AGE LIMIT FOR DONATIONS.** Besides organs, doctors can transplant skin for burn victims, corneas for vision and veins for blood flow. According to UNOS, United Network for Organ Sharing: as of October 12, 2017, the national list of people waiting for organ donations included:

Kidney	96,545
Liver	14,133
Pancreas	907
Kidney / Pancreas	1,684
Heart	3,979
Lung	1,355
Heart / Lung	42
Intestine	272

Others use religion as an argument. In my opinion, whatever the source, God, Buddha, or Allah, I believe in a higher power that bestows doctors/surgeons with the ability to perform life-saving surgeries. I'm thankful that my God gave my doctor the knowledge to perform the transplant. I'm confident other recipients will agree. My bumper sticker reads, *"Don't take your organs to heaven. Heaven knows we need them here."*

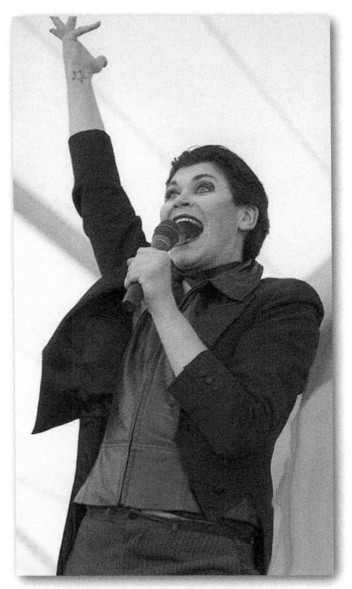

Adam Carter had the most energetic and flamboyant personality.

Chapter 11
CABARET

I'm offering the perspective from a donor family by sharing Adam Carter's story. He was a friend and amazing talent and, sadly, he left us too soon.

With flair and aplomb, his ensemble was already planned for the big day. The movie *Do You Believe?* had wrapped up in March of 2015 and Adam Carter would be making his premier walk on the red carpet. A native of Kalamazoo, he was ecstatic to be returning to L.A. for the big event.

Then tragedy struck. On February 6th he suffered severe brain trauma as the result of a fatal tumble down the stairs in his home.

Adam Carter was well known in the Kalamazoo community as an actor, director, make-up artist, hairstylist and female impersonator. He had the most energetic and flamboyant personality. Along with style and confidence, he was always the life of the party, the star of the show. According to his sister, Kara Pelfresne, her brother was, *"A born entertainer. I'm surprised he didn't come out of the womb doing jazz hands.*

However, Adam was confident without being arrogant. He could walk into a large crowd and be the most captivating person in the room. Everyone would remember Adam and talk of him for years."

Adam's mother, Terri Pelfresne offers her perception of the events.

As a result of his fall, Adam had multiple skull fractures and broken bones. Unresponsive when we reached him, we made the 911 call. As a mother it was something I never expected to do. I could hardly contain my tears as Bill and I drove behind the ambulance to the hospital. Upon arrival, not knowing I wasn't supposed to be in there, I followed the gurney into the triage room.

The lead doctor was amazing to watch, cutting off his clothes and giving orders. I heard her say, "his pupils are blown." It was then that someone approached me and said, "It would be better if you went to the waiting room to be with your husband." I didn't want to leave my Adam.

My two sisters arrived immediately. Our daughter Kara was driving in from Chicago. She only knew he had fallen, no details. When the doctor spoke to us, he revealed that in twenty minutes after arriving, because of the severity of his skull fractures, Adam would be brain dead.

Shock set in. What? How can that be? How would you know so soon? Are you sure? Brain dead? Are you sure? This is a kid who is overflowing with life. This can't be true.

Always the same answer, yes.

When Kara arrived, she had no idea what news was awaiting her. When her dad and I told her, she looked at me and said, "Mom, no, it can't be, are they sure? How do they know?" The same questions we'd asked before. With the waiting room empty at that time of night, it was easier to cry, to question, to hug, and to disbelieve.

When we finally saw him in the ER, his face, nostrils, and ears were bloody and had only been given a quick wipe at that time. He was then moved to the seventh floor. Because our group increased, we were given a staff room to wait. We were all praying and trying to let what happened sink in.

Some support came when we met a wonderful man from the Gift of Life Michigan. Having been through this many times, he knew what we were experiencing. He explained the options and the benefits of organ donation. We were able to ask questions of him and the two other Gift of Life volunteers. Concerning potential recipients, they could only tell us limited details due to confidentiality. We felt an overwhelming appreciation for, and from them. Care and concern radiated from the entire staff.

When they led us to Adam's room on the seventh floor he had been cleaned up. No remnants of his tragic fall were visible. He appeared to be sleeping, ready to awaken and break into a song at any minute. Holding his hands, we caressed him, kissed his face and showered him with expressions of our love.

In the staff room, which I called the "war room," a battle was raging that we were sure to lose. Food and drinks were brought to us for our vigil. One sister called to alert family and friends. Another sister sat by Adam's side for all but two hours of this ordeal. Kara was in charge of the social media end.

We set up a "Go Fund Me" page for Adam's love, the Kalamazoo Council for the Arts. Through the gifts of family and friends we raised a significant amount of money . . . over $15,000. We were not familiar with many who donated, but they indicated they were recipients as well. He would have been so proud. We were.

When the family realized it was time to speak with the Gift of Life volunteers again, Bill, Kara, and I made the decision to give his heart, liver, kidneys, and both lungs. Adam was a loving and giving person. We knew in our hearts he would have wanted it that way. When I asked about potential recipients, they could only reveal limited information.

We were told that five people would benefit from Adam's donation . . . three people were in critical condition and "close by." We assumed that meant in Kalamazoo at either Bronson or Borgess Hospitals. Another recipient was in Michigan, but the location was not disclosed. The fifth patient was out of the state.

For each one of the recipients there were three doctors in the operating room at the time of the surgery. Per the hospital's request, we had written some background information about Adam to be read preceding the operation. With the reading complete, there was a moment of silence. A spiritual energy enveloped the room and it was amazing he was honored in that way. We were touched with the empathy from everyone involved. I will never forget that feeling as long as I live.

From Bill Pelfresne:

> *Terri mentioned how the Gift of Life asked for a statement with personal details about Adam. It was to be read aloud before doctors began harvesting organs. They do this to humanize the donor and show how much he was loved.*
>
> *But Terri left something out in her description. After reading the letter she and Kara had written, she started out the door. We never thought she would relinquish Adam so easily. As they were coming to remove him from life support, Terri suddenly stopped. She desperately insisted that someone find a dark red lipstick for her. Before we could run to the store, a nurse appeared with the appropriate item. Terri lifted the shade to her lips, and Adam left the room on the seventh floor with his mother's red kiss on the center of his forehead. To the surgeons, that imprint said more than anyone could ever write.*

All five organs were donated, and the recipients are doing well. What more could we have asked? A loss was turned into a positive experience. Five families were given more time with their loved ones. We are so glad for Gift of Life. Their knowledge and compassion made all of us feel honored to do this for others.

Another gift that Adam left us was an increase in our Gift of Life donor list. After witnessing the events, many of his friends and family became registered donors. Still, there is a great need for more. Please contact them at donatelife.net and sign up today.

Through the Gift of Life Michigan staff/volunteers and by the grace of God, we were able to help. Our gratitude to them and to the staff on the seventh floor of Borgess Hospital for their care and concern.

~ The Family of Adam F. Carter~

Michigan residents can contact the Gift of Life at www.giftoflifemichigan.org.

After my surgery, I joined several social media sites for lung transplant survivors. I friended John Shea, a young man who posted some remarkable advice on how he faced the fact that surgery was not a guarantee of survival. He wrote this brilliant piece which I share it with his permission:

"As we are all aware, transplant surgery is long, intense, and probably the riskiest thing we have had to do. But at least for me, there were no options. I could go on "living" an extremely limited life, or I could take a chance at a new life. A life, not without challenges, but one at least where I could breathe and start planning for a future. I was conscious of how worried my family was about the surgery. There was a possibility that I could die. But I came to peace with that because I knew without the transplant I wouldn't live.

I did something that helped me through the waiting process and I'd like to share it with you. Once I was placed on the transplant list, I started writing letters to all of my family and friends. Letters I wanted them to read if I didn't make it through the surgery. I told them how much I loved and appreciated them. I told them how they positively affected my life. I also told them good-bye and that I didn't, and wouldn't regret opting for the surgery. I wanted to make sure that if I wasn't going to see them again, they knew how special they were to me. I gave all the sealed letters to my best friend. I left some money for postage and instructed her to mail them to everyone if I didn't survive.

Well I made it! On my one-year transplant anniversary I decided to mail the letters. It was probably the most rewarding thing I have ever done.

So, my advice is to find peace in both outcomes and do what you need to do to get through the process without regrets."

One of the most interesting books I've read on organ recipients is **The Heart's Code** by Dr. Paul Pearsall. He has collected an array of anecdotal material from organ transplant patients and their families. He claims that in many heart recipients, a spiritual tie grows between patient and donor. Some of the people interviewed claim to share memories with their deceased donors.

The theory has been proven in lung transplant patients as well. One incident I remember reading about was a woman who hated peanut butter before her surgery and craved it after the operation. Unfortunately, I haven't experienced this phenomenon. I think it would be fascinating.

In 2016, Rich and I decided to explore our DNA through Ancestry. com. Curious whether my foreign lungs would alter the results, we contacted them through e-mail. We were surprised when they responded by saying, "It should not be an issue." I found that difficult to believe, but when the results returned, there were no surprises according to the outcome. I had been told all my life, I was English, Irish, Scottish with some Scandinavian. And that's exactly what the report disclosed.

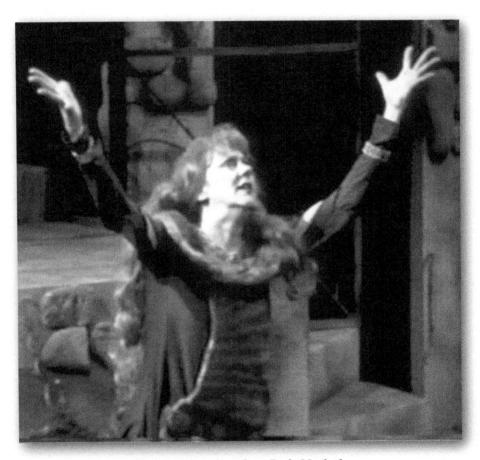

One of my favorite roles – Lady Macbeth.

Chapter 12
THE TEMPEST

Consuming massive doses of medication wreak havoc on your body. Even though I didn't have a choice, I was embarrassed that I had to wear Depends way before the transplant. On one occasion, I was in a big box store with a cart partly filled and all of a sudden it happened—that rumbling sensation down below. I walked briskly—running was not in my vocabulary—to the nearest bathroom. A loaded adult diaper is not pleasant, and walking seemed to encourage the "movement." Another time I was in St. Croix at the beach, and it all landed in my bathing suit, so I was able to take that off, clean it out and put my pants back on commando style. I no longer have to don the plastic panties. Thank God.

In December of 2009, we drove to U of M to ascertain what was happening with my bowels. In another episode to challenge my dignity, I had to choke down some chalky, nasty-tasting barium for an X-ray. The male nurse handed me the best set up line: "Just hold it in your mouth until I tell you to swallow." My mind immediately went to the naughty place and the comedienne in me wanted to say, "If I had a nickel for every time I've heard that," but I was good. I said nothing.

One night in the hospital, let's just say the brown river was churning. A nurse came into my room and politely asked if Brian could help with cleaning me up. Brian was a cute, mid-twenties technician with gorgeous eyes. "Well, hell yes," I said. "That would be the most excitement I've had in years." While they were doing their duty, I started groaning and told him a little to the left, a little to the right, higher, lower. When he finished, I asked for a cigarette and told Brian, "You can clean me anytime. How about tomorrow?" I guess I scared the poor kid off because his face turned beet red and made a mad dash for the door, never to be seen again.

After many episodes of uncooperative bowels, my doctor prescribed a new medication. I went from running bowels to constipation. Now some of you may have had some constipation, but this was **CONSTIPATION** that doubled me over in pain. When it didn't improve, I was taken to the local hospital by ambulance and I was given a series of enemas. Lovely, right? When those didn't work and after more hours of agony, I was transported by ambulance to the U of M hospital. Every single bump in the road jolted my body with unbearable pain.

When we arrived, they prescribed a gallon of "Go Lightly" and ordered me to drink the whole jug in an hour. Okay, the name slayed me. In the first place this was not *Breakfast at Tiffany's*. I told the doctors, "I can't even drink a gallon of something I like, let alone something that tastes like month-old cabbage." And the name, well, I didn't want to go lightly, I wanted to go abundantly and get that shit out of me. Pun intended. I was able to drink about two twelve oz. cups before I would start vomiting. I was thinking, oh, sure, I can puke but I can't poop.

But the epitome of bowel blockage was the day Dr. "I"—whom I had never seen before—came into my room. When he started putting on rubber gloves, I knew I was in trouble. He said, "I want to take a look at what's going on," and proceeded to shove his finger up my rear end. The pain was so excruciating I thought I was going to fly off the bed. Without thinking, my hand immediately went into action and with all the strength of Wonder Woman, I whacked him on the arm. Astounded, he jumped off the bed and just stared at me. "I was only trying to . . ." "That freakin' hurt," I screamed. I told him to get out of my room and he was not to touch me again. Stunned, he left. However, the next day Dr. "I" came back. What was he thinking? The minute he stepped in the door I said, "You will not touch me." He tried to argue, but I stuck to my guns. After that I asked for and was assigned another, gentler doctor.

Nothing was working and I became increasingly anxious. Ultimately, they decided to insert a tube through my nose, down into my stomach, so they could pump in the liquid goo. Since it was so painful, it took two nurses to hold me down. When the tubing touched the back of my throat, my gaging reflex hit the limit. I happened to catch the reflection of what was happening in the window and I continued gagging, but trying to laugh at the same time. The muddy reflection looked like an ancient sex ritual or a scene from a Three Stooges movie. They finally positioned it to the correct spot, but I could feel it touching the back of my throat. It remained there for seven days.

When they had finished their business and left the room, mind wandered back to the torture chambers Rich and I had seen in English and Scottish castles. On release from the persecution, we discovered the bowel blockage was caused by the medication I was taking, and once again, my meds were changed.

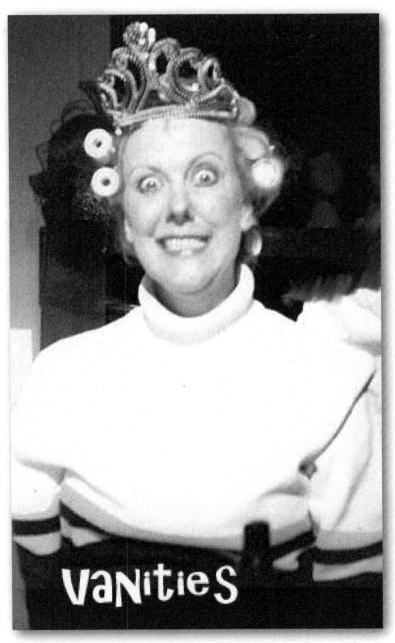

Pre-show goofiness for Vanities

Chapter 13
BEYOND THERAPY

Depression hit hard after the 2009 episode with bowels. If I couldn't get up fast enough, which was 9.9 out of 10 times, the brown goo streamed out of my bottom onto the couch and the floor. I never seemed to be in the bathroom when it happened—no such luck. I felt sorry for Rich because he had to clean me up every time. I just didn't have the strength. Then the vomiting ensued non-stop, and again, wherever I was because I couldn't move fast enough to get to the bathroom.

I've made light of my situation because it was the only way I could get through it. But I haven't told you about the dark side. There were many occasions when I wanted to give up. Ordinarily, not my nature, but because of all that was happening to me, I was spent.

Before the transplant, I was one of the pillars in the Kalamazoo the-atre community. As described in earlier chapters, I worked as the executive assistant and publicist for the Kalamazoo Civic Theatre business office for sixteen years. I performed and directed many productions there.

My life revolved around the theatre. I would work for eight hours in the office, go home for dinner, and then go back to the theatre for rehearsals—either directing or acting. I taught and partici-pated in classes on auditioning and acting.

In the 1980's, I was a member of the New Vic Theatre, and for ten years, my murder mystery company, *Suspenders*, was in full swing.

The point of all this is to illustrate how, for many years, I was defined by my career. Because I worked in the heart of the local theatre scene—the Civic business office—I knew many volunteers and many patrons. People respected me because of my career. My identity was completely defined by my role in the theatre. My life was creating fantasy.

And then reality stepped in.

In 2007, I had to leave my job at the Civic due to poor health. And from 2008 to 2009, after the transplant, my entire life was dedicated to resolving precarious health issues. I was once known as a hot, funny, sexy broad, but I gained thirty pounds resulting in large doses of Prednisone. I also developed the dreaded spare tire, which remains with me as of this writing. UGH. And along with that drug came *Cushingoid*, which I referred to it as puff-fish face. [+11]

I was in and out of the hospital hanging onto life by my fingernails. For that reason, I became defined by my illness and my weakness. Because of my limited mobility and compromised immune system, I was unable to attend the theatre, let alone participate in a production. I wanted to be a good friend by supporting the people I cared about. I wanted to be, as before, someone who could be counted on. But I had no control over this malady. I never knew from one day to the next how I was going to feel and I felt guilty because my friends couldn't depend on me. I was always apologizing for something that wasn't my fault.

I felt like I was drowning and no one was throwing out a life preserver. I compared my long illness to a death . . . in the beginning, friends brought casseroles, cards, and flowers, but after a while they stopped coming. Of course, everyone has their own lives and their own issues, but I was so damned angry that this was my lot. I started to feel abandoned and lonely. In a drug-induced haze, I lashed out and wrote a nasty letter to two of my best friends. Everything I wrote was my truth, my insecurity. It was a cry for help. It was my perception of my horrific situation. Unfortunately, as much as I apologized, it wasn't their truth. It was hurtful, and it distressed me to know that I was responsible for destroying our wonderful relationships. They both suffered unthinkable tragedies and I was able to help a little, but from then on, all of our lives had changed.

After two years of constant pain, two years of endless worry for my husband, daughter, and family, I went into a debilitating depression that was completely foreign to me. We were, after all, the fun family. I hit rock bottom and I didn't want to continue living that way.

One night, while in the hospital, the pain medication wasn't working. I was in so much agony and close to losing consciousness. Slurring my words, I said to Rich, "I don't want to do this anymore. I don't want to go on if all I have to look forward to are daily health issues. This is not life. I'm done."

Rich came over and sat on the bed. He lifted my chin and with tears in his eyes said, "Please don't leave me."

How could I give up when his love inspired me? It took a long time to convince me. But even if I couldn't do it for me, I had to find a way to live for Rich's sake.

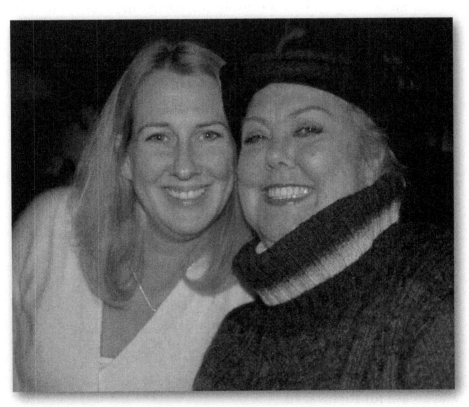

Susan and her chipmunk mother.

Chapter 14
TRAVESTIES

With every clinic visit, Dr. Chan would ask me, "Was it worth it?" For the longest time, I couldn't say yes. There was too much pain. Too much life being wasted and passing me by as I became one with the couch. It was such a long time to be sedentary. I felt restless and most of all useless.

2010, a couple of years after the transplant, I started to feel better. My lung function was up and I was finally released from my oxygen leash. Wheezy had to go back to her own home. Even though she'd been my constant companion, I was ecstatic when they came to pick her up.

One morning I was walking down the stairs with a spring in my step and with surprising ease. I stopped. So, this is what it's like to feel normal again? After two years I felt as if I had regained my life. In 2012 Rich and I celebrated our fortieth anniversary by travelling to Trinidad and Tobago for a tropical get away. I directed *Nunsense* at the Marshall Civic Theatre and *The Foreigner* for the Kalamazoo Civic. I auditioned for and was cast in one of my coveted roles - the nurse in *Romeo and Juliet*. And a few months later I performed in the highly acclaimed *33 Variations*. An amazing script written by Moises Kaufman. The play addresses Beethoven's obsession with Diabelli's waltz. I received the *Excellence in Performance Award* for the role of Gertie in that production. Needless to say, I made up for those lost two years.

I must have overdone it because in June 2012, just after *33 Variations* closed, my body started rejecting my new lungs. I was transported to Ann Arbor via ambulance and spent the next month in the hospital.

REJECTION. One the most dreaded words for actors, but the most terrifying word for organ recipients. Actors and actresses develop tough skin by experiencing rejection many times in their careers. In community theatre, at least ten actors audition for the same role. I'm confident that for Broadway, movies, and TV there are hundreds. The director and producer must decide who exemplifies the role and, most importantly, who fits in with the cast as a whole. She/he has only x number of roles to fill, so many hopeful actors will be disappointed. I am all too familiar with that kind of rejection.

In June of 2012, four years after my surgery, I experienced a different kind of rejection. The life-threatening kind. My body said, "Hey, what are these unidentified flying wind bags doing in here?" I was experiencing cold like symptoms for about two weeks. I let it go that long because I was exasperated with hospital and doctor visits. I didn't think it was serious enough to make an appointment for a couple of sniffles. I was due for a checkup at U of M, so I decided to wait. Bad idea.

From the very beginning of this medical mystery tour I was warned that if I went into rejection, any loss of lung function was permanent and could be fatal. I had no idea that these were the signs of rejection. Or maybe subconsciously, I didn't want to know.

We made the trip to Ann Arbor and without hesitation they admitted me into the hospital. To say we were astonished would be putting it mildly. Up until that point I had been feeling great. I was acting, directing, swimming. We were travelling again. I hadn't been hospitalized in three years and, optimistically, we thought all of my medical issues were over.

Rich had to work the next day, so he felt horrible when he had to leave me there. But he didn't need to see me in any more pain. His job was stressful enough.

They began treating me for rejection but we discovered later they weren't sure what was happening. I was put on 700mg of Prednisone along with some other medications. I had two transfusions and I was put back on oxygen. I also went through a process called Plasma Apheresis - *"a method of removing blood plasma from the body, separating it into plasma and cells, and transfusing the cells back into the bloodstream. It is performed to remove antibodies in treating auto-immune conditions."*

Even with all the infusions and transfusions, nothing seemed to work, so they began treating me for pneumonia. I was in the hospital for twenty-seven days. Even though I hated it, my body was telling me I needed to be there. There is an unwritten rule that for every day you're in the hospital, it takes three days to recover. So, after this stint, I would be facing eighty-one days of recuperation. After learning this theory, I became increasingly depressed.

During that time, I couldn't keep anything down. That was problematic because I needed to eat before I took my medication. Two doctors were chastising me to take my meds, and I screamed at them, "If I can't freakin' breathe, and I can't freakin' eat, how am I supposed to take my freakin' pills?" The next day I apologized for my behavior. One doctor sat down and very gently told me that he understood my frustration. He explained they weren't sure what was happening, so they were trying different procedures to cover all the bases. And because they had increased the doses of all medication, it was making me sick. I was so appreciative of his candor and I wished more doctors would establish his bedside manner.

With that tiny piece of knowledge, I felt assured and a little more trust. I was finally able to choke down the pills.

The good news was, for whatever reason, I pulled through it. To this day, the doctors scratch their heads and wonder why I'm still alive. They call me their miracle patient. I loved how one nurse phrased it, "You must have some hefty angels watching over you."

The bad news was that because the rejection had caused scar tissue in my lungs, Wheezy had to come home with me indefinitely. As luck would have it, I only needed two LPM and if I sat still, my levels would stay at 94 - 97. However, when I got up to move, the LPM would drop to 83 - 87. Needless to say, a 5K was not in my future.

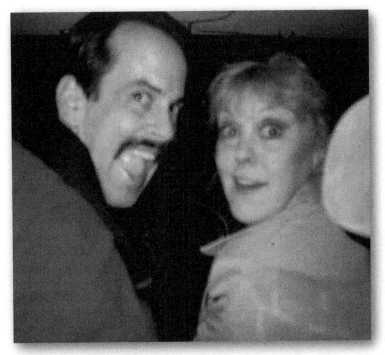

The fun family on another exciting vacation.

Chapter 15
WIT

Whenever I am admitted to the hospital there is a faction of the staff who love to see me, and the other half who cringe when they learn I am to be their patient. Not that I'm rude or demanding, but by now you understand I speak up when I feel something isn't acceptable. I truly believe that nurses are saints. I don't understand how they can witness pain and suffering every day. I try to maintain my sense of humor not only for my benefit, but to offer some levity for the nurses and doctors as well, even if it's only for a few minutes. This chapter is a compilation of such moments as anecdotes, incidents, and observations during the many hours spent in institutions of medicine.

Susan
There was the time I took my mom to a check-up appointment. She was very weepy. Complaining about the doctors, complaining about the meds, complaining about her life. I think this was in February of 2009. I had recently experienced losing my father-in-law to cancer and a tragedy occurred on our street where a seven-year old neighbor boy had been run over by a truck while sledding down his hill. He died at the end of my driveway and I witnessed it. Too tragic to talk about. Let's just say my compassion meter for my mom was not on the high end. I told her to, "Get used to it. This is her life and she should be thankful she is here experiencing the doctors and the pills." I don't think she knows why I snapped at her - until she reads this flash of memory. We joke about it now and call it GUTI.

THE WEIR: I was complaining about some infirmity when Susan replied G.U.T.I. "What the heck is *guti?*" I questioned. She adamantly replied, "Get Used to It." I almost used it for the title of this book.

BOEING, BOEING: One particular occasion while we were travelling, the security agent took my portable oxygen device to scan. It was taking a long time because they were busy with other passengers. Finally, in my best Bronx accent, I choked out, "Hey, I'm dyin' here." They got the message and quickly handed it back.

RUMORS: When any medical course of action must be done, my doctor proceeds with caution. He explains, "You're not normal." I respond, "Well, it is rumored that that is true, but it's too late to change my ways."

THE SOUND OF MUSIC: During one procedure I was assigned a very good looking young African American intern. He had what I describe as "a three balls voice." When he spoke, the sound resonated in this deep, delicious baritone. I deemed him the Barry-White-Wannabe, but in a good way. At first, I wondered if he would be offended, but when he broke out into a deep, rumbling chuckle, I knew it was okay. I kept begging him to sing "*Can't Get Enough of Your Love Baby.*"

OUT CRY: Taking blood gases was one of the most excruciating procedures I have had to endure, not once, not twice, but three times. Trust me when I say it is painful. It felt as though someone was sticking needles under my fingernails, only this was happening in my wrist. Said wrist would be strapped down to the bedside table to complete the procedure. The nurse was quite thorough in cleaning and explained, "I have to make sure your hand is exceptionally clean." To which I replied, "Well of course you do. You don't know where it's been." He gave me a funny look "Whaaaa?" "Never mind," I said.

MORNING'S AT SEVEN: The 7:00am nurse was pushing me to take my meds. I told her I had to have something in my stomach before I could do so. She continued to implore. As she was a sweet young thing, I complied. So, what do you suppose happened? Spewing vomit. "For my next magical trick . . ." I said. Not only was she embarrassed that she hadn't listened to me, but she was perturbed when she had to clean it up.

CRIMES OF THE HEART: On another day, my husband was in the room when a nurse sashayed in to adjust my oxygen. While she fiddled with the machine an alarm went off. With a quick wink to my husband, I grabbed my throat and began coughing and choking. The look on the nurse's face was priceless. When Rich burst out laughing, the nurse slapped me playfully and shrieked, "Don't ever do that again."

PROOF: There was a young technician from Manchester, England. As he prepared me for surgery, he asked, "Have you had anything to eat today?" I donned my best British accent and said, "No, I haven't and quite frankly, I'm a bit peckish." He was gob-smacked and shouted, "Where are you from?" Still "in character" I told him he had to guess. After several attempts, I went back to my nasally Midwest accent and said, "Actually, I'm from Kalamazoo, Michigan. He was really surprised that I had fooled him. I told him when I studied with The Royal National Theatre in London, one of our assignments was to infiltrate the city, strike up a conversation, and see if anyone could detect our secret. He thought that was fascinating. Unfortunately, I never saw him again. He told me he was moving to Arizona. I hope he likes it as much as we did.

KISMET: Then there was the male technician who was so sweet. He drew a beautiful rose on my "to do" board and teasingly said, "You know, I don't do this for everyone." Two years later, when I was admitted for procedure number 486, (sic), the same guy walked into my room. "Will you draw another rose for me?" I asked. He

couldn't believe I remembered him. He thought it was a small ges-
ture, but that little act of kindness meant so much to me.

SHE STOOPS TO CONQUER: On one visit to the emergency
room, Dr. "J" came in and began speaking to Rich, never making
eye contact with me. This went on for a few minutes until I finally
said, "Excuse me, I'm the patient here. Perhaps you'd better talk
to me." I don't know why that seemed like a new concept to him,
but he had difficulty with it.

BYE BYE BIRDIE: When you need to go to other areas of the
hospital, they don't just take you there, they "transport" you. The
nurse makes a call and someone comes, eventually, with either a
wheelchair or a gurney. Many times, they will just wheel you in
your bed. After a long stint in the ICU, they were transporting me,
in my bed, to a private room. Hooked up to IV's and a catheter
bag with an oxygen cannula in my nose, I looked like a monster
from one of those B horror movies. While we were rolling down
the hall, many of the staff were congratulating me on my recovery
and at one point I sat up and screamed, "**IT'S ALIVE.**"

On another occasion, when it was difficult for me to lie on my
back, I decided to sit up on the gurney for the whole ride. But, as
you can tell by now, that wasn't enough for me; I wrapped my blan-
kets around my shoulders and proceeded to emulate the Queen. I
had her down pat, complete with wave, the head turn, the touching of the pearls, while uttering, "Thank you my little people."

On one wheel-chair excursion, I told the transporter to go as fast
as he could down a long hall. He was afraid he would get in trouble, but I convinced him. I held both arms up and shouted E-ticket
ride . . . wheeeeeeeeeeeeeeee.

NINE: When the universal question regarding pain . . . on a scale
of one to ten was asked, I would always say fourteen.

THE DROWSY CHAPERONE: I would often ask Dr. Chan to write a prescription for me for medical marijuana—not to smoke, but for cookies or brownies. I wanted to re-live the 60's and 70's. He just laughed.

I was drinking a coke when someone told me about Mary Jane Gummy Bears. Not being able to contain my laugh, I did an enormous spit-take. I'm glad some states have legalized this drug. I have a friend in the early stages of Parkinson's disease and it helps ease the pain.

FUNNY GIRL: I pulled the old Vaudeville joke on one doctor. I asked, "Will I be able to play the piano after this?" "Oh, of course," the doctor said. "Well, that's funny, I never could before." RIMSHOT.

ON A CLEAR DAY: If you've ever had surgery, and been in a recovery room, you may have experienced this as well. When the nurse wakes you up they want to see how alert you are by posing various questions. In my case it went like this.

What's your name?	Cathie Weir
What year is it?	2009
Who's the president?	Obama
Where are you?	HELL

GREY GARDENS: When any bodily fluids erupted from one place or another, the question was always asked, "What color is it?" I couldn't just answer yellow or brown, no, I'd come up with something like, "A delicate shade of sage," or "banana yellow."

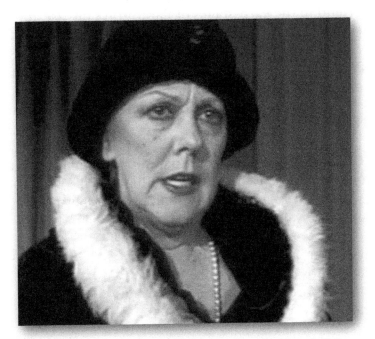

Another favorite Shakespeare role – Paulina in Winter's Tale.

Chapter 16
LES MISÉRABLES

Saturday, January 19, 2013—just two days shy of my five-year lun-gaversary, and six months after rejection, I woke up in severe pain and could not move any portion of my body. The only things that didn't hurt were my eyelashes. When I'm in pain, I don't scream like a lady. No, I grunt like a Neanderthal. And on that day, the entire tribe was chanting.

Rich rushed in and I blurted out, "Call 911." The twenty questions began: "What's wrong? Where's the pain on a scale of 1 - 10?" etc. I screeched, "Call the freakin' ambulance, I can't move." He decided to call Susan instead. Why? I can't tell you, but she was there in fifteen minutes. They struggled to get me dressed, helped me downstairs and we drove to a place all too familiar, the emergency room at Bronson, our local hospital.

The diagnosis was a perforated bowel, but no indication of how it might have happened was given. However, a nurse said that popcorn was often the perpetrator. Sure enough, we had some the night before with our Friday night movie.

Given my lack of immune system and complicated medical history, the Bronson team would frequently defer to U of M Hospital. The staff at Bronson would stabilize me until I was able to travel, often by ambulance. But given the gravity of the situation, they decided to airlift me. Forgetting the pain, I thought how exciting. I get to ride in a helicopter. I'd flown in one before and I loved it. To transfer me from the bed to the gurney, I was pulled up using the sheet method . . . a practice I was accustomed to. Two nurses on opposite sides of the bed each grabbed the sheet. They counted: one, two, and on the count of three, lifted the sheet up and moved me over to the "chariot." There was pain from being lifted, pain when they strapped me onto the rock-hard rescue board, and pain when they put me on the gurney. Okay, I thought, this might not be so much fun after all.

Rich asked the pilot, and the male nurse accompanying me, if he could ride with them. (I should mention that said nurse was a blond-haired, blue-eyed Adonis). Obviously, they said no, regulations and such. That's when Rich pulled his ace in the hole by whipping out his airport badge, "I'm an air traffic controller." And just like that he was in the door along for the ride. (Pilots respect controllers. Rich and his team receive compliments daily for their work.) I could hear my hubby inviting the pilot and Adonis to visit the tower for a private tour whenever they wanted. I was thinking, hey, this isn't a party, guys. Remember me, back here in pain? But they kept chatting away like long lost friends. In hindsight, it was good for Rich to get his mind off of what was in store.

It was January. It was Michigan. It was bitterly cold. I remember being on the roof, on the helipad and hearing the whoosh, whoosh of the chopper blades. The pain meds had set in and I was officially in la la land. Adonis said a couple of things and all I could do was drool. I don't know why I thought I had to be charming in that state, but it's just in my nature to flirt. Rich is the same way. Adonis fiddled around with the IV and after that I passed out. The next day I was disappointed because I had taken a helicopter ride and wasn't able to enjoy it. Rich revealed, "It was probably a good thing you were out. The flight was quite bumpy. We are seasoned travelers, but like everyone else, I get a little nervous when it's choppy. The drive to Ann Arbor from Kalamazoo is about two hours, but because of the tail winds, they made it in record time . . . twenty-one minutes.

I don't remember arriving, but Rich conveyed that once there, I was rushed in for emergency surgery. I woke up with a plastic bag hanging from the left side of my stomach. A tender vertical scar, two inches above my belly-button, ran down above my hairline. Doctors and nurses kept arriving asking if it was working. "What? What working?" What are you talking about?" They explained that when I have a BM, it would collect in the bag. Okay? I was completely clueless as to what was happening.

A nurse arrived laden with unrecognizable paraphernalia. She told me she was going to teach me how to change the colostomy bag. The conversation went something like this:

Me	Why would I need to know that?
Nurse	Well, it needs to be cleaned out whenever you have a BM.
Me	Isn't that the nurse's job?
Nurse	Well, from now on . . .
Me	Wait a minute. Are you telling me this is permanent?
Nurse	(To my husband) Didn't anyone tell her?
Rich	No.
Me	Tell me what?
Nurse	You'll be doing this at home.
	And then it dawned on me.
Me	You mean I'll have this for the rest of my life?

When the nurse nodded yes, I started sobbing uncontrollably. Just six months before I faced rejection and could have died. I couldn't believe I was given one more health issue to deal with. She politely excused herself and left the room.

Enough time passed so the nurse came back in to teach me how to clean the "pouch of poop." I was really concerned that I wouldn't be able to swim with this new development. The nurse assured me that the flange, the part that sticks to your body, and the pouch were as water-tight as Tupperware. Now that made me laugh. So, we began the lesson. Let's not even mention the smell. I began cleaning it, making sure to get all the residual stuff out when she said, "You don't have to be so clean." My reply was "I know, but I'm <u>anal</u> about it." Not a flicker of recognition. Another one who didn't get my humor. Geez. Tough crowd.

This would be the perfect place to say if it wasn't for Rich, I wouldn't be here today. He has a way of soothing and comforting me during difficult times. And we have had many: losing our parents, scraping by on minimum wages, and countless moves. He can take any negative situation and turn it into a positive one. But this was one of the toughest.

I was imprisoned in the University of Michigan Hospital for two weeks. Now U of M is a teaching hospital and you have the right to allow or deny onlookers. I had no problem with it because modesty was another word not in my vocabulary. In the theatre when you need to make a quick costume change, there's no time to be self-conscious. Actors are backstage waiting to make their entrances and they'll do nothing short of a striptease to make their cue. Theatre folk have been accused of being exhibitionists. That's not far from the truth. Both on and off stage.

During those two weeks, a new cast of characters entered my story. Most memorable was Dr. "K" the Ice Princess. She was thirty-something, small in stature, pretty, but all business. She strolled into the room with six interns following her like the mice trailing the Pied Piper. She drew up my gown and explained to me, "I'm going to stick my finger into your wound to see how deep it is."

It was one of the most perfect set up lines I had ever heard, and I couldn't let it pass by. "Well, I'm usually taken to dinner before that happens, AND I expect to be kissed." The six followers exploded in laughter, but Dr. Ice Princess didn't crack a smile, no expression whatsoever. "What did you say?" she finally asked. So, I repeated it. She replied, "I thought that's what you said." I shot back, "Well, they all got it." When she abruptly left the room, I told the little mice, "Give her a quarter and tell her to go buy a sense of humor."

A year later the surgeon, Dr. "L," told me I could have the operation reversed and I could poop like normal people. GREAT. But there was a deal breaker. The reversal included two surgeries. I contemplated for a minute and then asked him if he could perform a tummy tuck while he was down there. When he declined, so did I. If I wasn't going to get Cher's waist, I wasn't going back to the hospital, let alone willingly. The whole ordeal was an education because I now know where the term "sack of s**t" comes from.

By the time I recovered from the bowel blockage, it was 2014. All in all, it was a good year. Other than regular checkups, I didn't have to see the inside of a hospital. I was extremely happy about that.

The best year I've had since my surgery was 2015. In January, we traveled to Clearwater, Florida, and met up with long lost friends. February found us in Phoenix where I saw cousins I hadn't seen in forty-five years. We went to Chicago twice, once for Rich's birthday. We rode the Ferris wheel on Navy Pier, and sailed on Windy to watch the fireworks over Lake Michigan. The second time was to see *The Lion King*. In November, we travelled to Curacao with Susan, her beau, Aaron, and our granddaughter Hannah. I watched my daughter and granddaughter swim with the dolphins while I had the less-interactive "dolphin encounter." We sailed on the Galaxie (the three-hour tour) and the weather did get rough, but I loved it.

I performed in *Motherhood Out Loud* with some of my dearest friends. But the biggest thrill was receiving the *Community Medal of Arts Award*, the most prestigious arts award in Kalamazoo. I was there when my granddaughter turned thirteen. I was also able to attend many of her swim meets where she won first place ribbons.

I took two writing courses with Olli/WMU. And just the fact that I was able to do all that was miraculous.

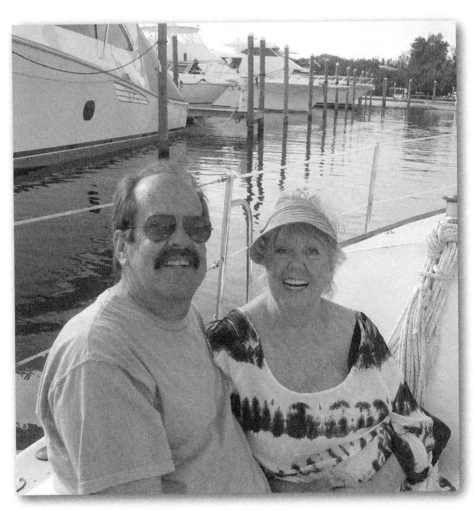

Boat ride in Anna Maria Island.

Chapter 17
A LESSON FROM ALOES

Even though I refer to hospitals as torture chambers, I'm quite confident that doctors don't wake up every morning rubbing their hands together with wide satanic eyes and in their best James Earl Jones' voice proclaim, "Ooooooooo, how many patients can I mutilate today?" There is going to be pain. Trust me. It's just the nature of the beast. You need to discover your way of dealing with it. I chose humor.

If it weren't for the doctors and nurses, I wouldn't be alive today. However, I know my own body. I know what will work for me and what won't. I hope everyone understands that it is acceptable to refuse a procedure or a medication. I have on several occasions. Especially when I was asked to participate in "study." I didn't want to be anyone's Guinea pig. What I was going through was difficult enough. I wasn't going to add anything that could compromise my already precarious health or cause more pain.

If you take away anything from this book, I hope it will be this: You have choices. Doctors and nurses, however brilliant, don't have all the answers. Some will even admit it. If you feel uncomfortable with a physician, look for another one. This also applies to caregivers. I was lucky enough to have family members who stepped in when I needed their help . . . others might not be as fortunate. Dealing with a serious illness is stressful for all involved: the patient, the family, and the caregiver. You need to trust the person who oversees your health and welfare. Something as simple as a personality conflict can create unnecessary stress. You have a voice, so use it to your advantage. If you feel unable to do so, hospitals provide patient advocates who will defend your rights and have your wishes honestly considered when decisions are being made about your life.

Something else I've discovered was that onlookers tend to praise the patient for surviving, while the caregivers go unnoticed. Caregivers often have it worse than the patient. They deserve some credit. They have to sit helplessly by and watch the pain and suffering. They are left to deal with their own silent grief about the situation, without the means to "fix" it. Their dedication and loyalty are above reproach, and they need a pat on the back every once in a while.

From my vantage point, as a patient, I'd like to offer friends and family something I've learned. Please don't give up on me. Please include me in activities. Don't automatically assume that I am unable to do something. I became so frustrated when people would ask me, "Are you healthy enough," or "Do you feel up to it?" I wished they would have asked, "How can I help you achieve your goals, or "What can I do to make things better for you?" For the patient, it puts a positive spin on a challenging situation.

There were times when I felt as though people were uncomfortable around me and as I've reported, I felt abandoned. I couldn't understand why people were behaving that way. Maybe I'm a reminder of their own mortality. Yes, I've had some major health issues, but I'm still here. I'm still laughing.

When I am out and about, I rarely see people sporting oxygen tanks. Individuals have confessed they wished their loved ones would be as "brave" as me. I don't consider myself brave at all. I didn't go through countless procedures or suffer indescribable pain to sit on the sidelines. I'm living on borrowed time and I'm going to make the most of it.

I know it's difficult, but I would like to encourage you to go out at least once a week, to the mall, the library or a park. If you have a special interest, many classes are available at libraries and universities. If you are over fifty, senior centers provide many beneficial services. You'll meet people with similar curiosities and, who knows, you might meet a new friend. Sitting at home all day can be debilitating and depressing. If you have limited mobility, check your local community for disabilities organizations or Senior Service Centers for FREE transportation.

I would also like to point out that mine is an exclusive story. If you are considering transplantation of any organ, please understand that all cases are different. When we were considering our options, we tried not to look at information on the internet. We didn't want to compare my situation with anyone else. There are transplant survivors who have lived unchallenged for twenty years. Then there are others who never make it off the operating table.

And please, more than anything else, go to donatelife.net, and sign up today to become a donor. It isn't enough to sign the back of your driver's license anymore, you need to register on line. With that done, make your wishes known to your family and friends should the need arise. When you become a donor, you become a potential hero.

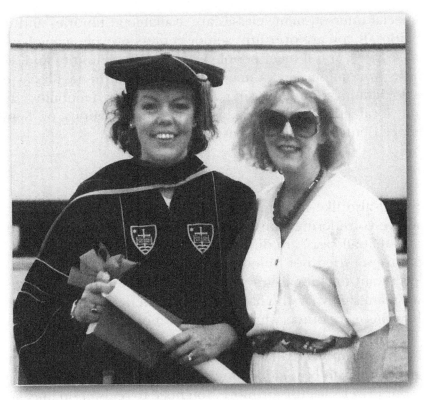

Rosemary receives her degree from Notre Dame.

Chapter 18
STEEL MAGNOLIAS

Accepting the limitations of my life is easier when I think about it from a spiritual perspective. I was, and still am a very strong woman with a strong voice. I wouldn't have made it through if I wasn't. Sometimes that voice wasn't used wisely. Maybe my karma was to tone it down a bit. I believe I'm a little kinder/gentler now. Before, when something infuriated me, I would have a knee jerk reaction and fly off the handle. Now I tend to weigh the pros and cons before making a judgement. Before I would tell people to raise their arms over their heads, with fingers touching to form a circle and say, "Here's the world. Find the problem." It's truer now more than ever.

I'm positive that survivors of tragedies feel the same way when they ask their God, "Why did you save me? What do you want me to do?" God hasn't answered my question yet. Maybe it was to write this book, I don't know. Maybe it was to point out the need to "stop and smell the roses." Or find joy in the simple things and cherish the moments you spend with the ones you love. I know that sounds cliché, but it's very true.

Because of my transplant, Rich and I have shared more anniversaries and travels. I've celebrated more birthdays with friends and family. I've seen my daughter find happiness with a new partner. I've seen my granddaughter grow from birth to the beautiful young lady she is today. As adults, Rosemary and I never lived in the same place at the same time. In 2013, she and Alan moved five miles away from us. We have developed a wonderful relationship by travelling, celebrating the holidays and sharing dinners. And what's really great is that all four of us, Rosemary, Alan, Rich and I are all compatible and we <u>reconnoiter</u> many adventures. (That one is for Alan!)

I've had an astonishing life. As Howard Carter exclaimed when he discovered King Tutankhamun's tomb, "I see wonderful things." Well, I have seen wonderful things: the Eiffel Tower, the Grand Canyon, the battlefields of Gettysburg, the Sistine Chapel, Michelangelo's David, the Coliseum, Mona Lisa, Arc de Triomphe, St. Paul's Cathedral, the Tower of London. I rode a hydrofoil from Hong Kong to China. I swam with the dolphins, rode a streetcar in San Francisco and swam in the Mediterranean and Caribbean Seas. Two of the most overwhelming experiences were visiting the Anne Frank House in Amsterdam, seeing her original diary and visiting the military cemetery at Normandy.

It has been *A Wonderful Life.*

In my dream, when my father said, "**I'll see you later,**" I interpreted it to mean that I was going to be okay and not to worry. Almost ten years later, I am doing just fine.

Susan

So, we had to get used to it. The trying times; the bumps in the road. There was a time I drove for five hours in a blizzard to get my mom out of the hospital. In normal conditions, it takes an hour and forty-five minutes to get to Ann Arbor. Cars swerving off the highway and spinning in my path – all I could think about was getting my mom out of there. I felt bad she had to wait so long for me to get there.

Watching my mom hurt and then watching my dad hurt just as much - seeing his love in pain has been . . . well, rough. There were times, I had to witness my strong dad weep. Breaks my heart...

My dad also went through some health issues. Mom wasn't able to be with him and I had to take him to U of M. Scary to see your parents weak and hurting.

But you know what? I would much rather go through all of these tribulations again, because if we hadn't - they wouldn't be here. We have been to Curacao, St. Martin, and Chicago for family trips. They have been great. I love my family. Next trips – Barbados and Anna Maria Island here we come.

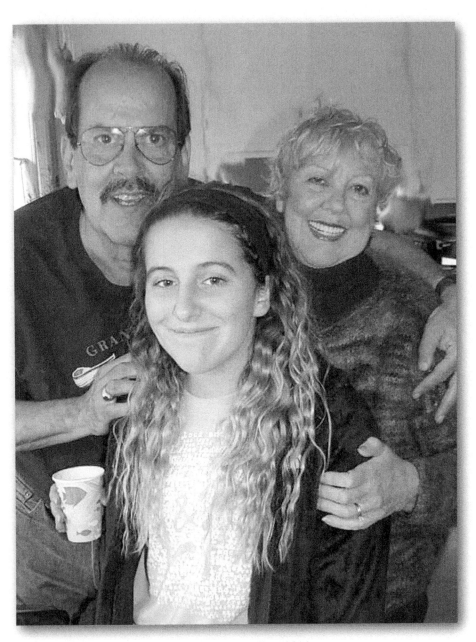

Rich, Hannah and me 2016.

Chapter 19
LOVE LETTERS

May 18, 2017
FOR MY SWEETIE.

I feel extremely lucky to have my wife Cathie with me to enjoy more years together. In 2007, we were told that without a lung transplant she only had a 20% chance of living another five years. With the transplant, her chances for survival went up to 80%.

She went through a full year of tests before she qualified and was put on the transplant list. Not long afterward, a transplant team was coming back from Milwaukee with lungs for another patient waiting at the University of Michigan Hospital. The jet crashed and killed all on board. It was a horrible tragedy, not only for the U of M staff, but for the patient waiting for those lungs. It may sound selfish, but I was afraid that with the loss of the transplant team, her chances of getting a new set of lungs were slim. Somehow, our luck continued. Three months after she finished her testing we got a call telling us to get to the hospital because there was a possible donor.

When we arrived at the hospital, we were advised that the donor had not yet passed and we were to wait there. Hours later, we were told Cathie was to be prepped for surgery. Our daughter, Susan, came with us for moral support during the surgery. The doctors told me it would take a few hours and that if we wanted to, we could either wait there or leave. They would call us when the surgery was completed. We decided to leave, get something to eat, and get some rest. Staying at the hospital was not an option for me since I always try to be positive. Being there seemed like a death watch and I didn't want to do that.

After eight hours, we got a call from the doctor that surgery was complete, that it went well, and Cathie was in recovery and would be awake within about an hour. We went to the hospital and spoke to the doctor. At that time, the doctor told us she received two lungs. Again, very lucky, as we were warned earlier it was very likely that she would only get one lung. It was a scary sight to see all the wires and tubes attached to her.

We've had quite a few setbacks over the years, however, the best thing is that we're still together and able to travel and do other things we enjoy. I am looking forward to another ten years. Cathie gives me a lot of credit for helping her and being positive. I could not do it without her. She is my hero and my inspiration. I could never be as strong.

Your loving husband,
Rich

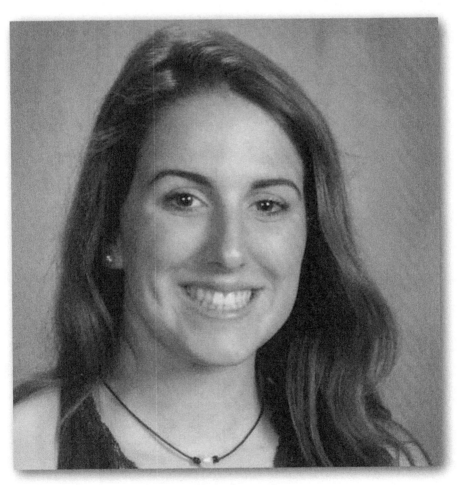

Hannah's freshman photo.

MY HERO, MY GRANDMA
by Hannah – 5th grade assignment

My Grandma, Cathie Weir, a caring woman, is my hero. She always remains positive, she is perseverant, and not to mention she is also very creative. Because of that, she is the best person I could write this paper about, the best wife a husband could ever ask for and the best mother a daughter could ever ask for. I am so thankful and lucky to have her love me unconditionally all the time.

My Grandma turns to me and lets out a sigh as she is delicately set into an old squeaky wheelchair at the Dolphin Academy. "No biggy," Grandma says as she smiles. "Do you want to walk?" my grandpa asks my grandma nicely. My grandma shakes her head no and continues getting pushed in the wheelchair.

Shortly my grandma is slowly immersed into the crystal-clear light blue water filled with silky gray dolphins. But not being able to swim with them, (she did that two years before), just 'meet' them. She pets the cute dolphins and has an ear to ear smile stretched across her face. My grandma is so positive throughout life and I find a lot of inspiration in how she finds the best in everything, and turns every bad situation into a good one.

My Grandma was diagnosed with a lung disease and had to have a very important surgery, a double lung transplant. A lung transplant is surgery to remove a person's diseased lung and replace it with a healthy lung from a deceased donor. But in her case, both of her lungs. Lung transplants are used for people who are likely to die from lung disease within one to two years. My grandma also has a nasal cannula. You see them in hospitals, movies like *The Fault in Our Stars*, or even TV, but I recognize them from my grandma. Basically, a nasal cannula is something to deliver oxygen or increase the airflow to a patient or person in need of respiratory help. It is a lightweight tube where one end splits into two nub like prongs which are placed in the nostrils and from which a mixture of air oxygen flows into the nose so they can breathe. I remember watching my grandma put it in her nose and take all her medications. Some days my grandma would have to give herself a shot. That would freak me out. My grandma would pick up the tiny syringe and I would squint my eyes not wanting to see her do it, but being my curious self, I would peek. She would insert the needle into her upper thigh and the vial of liquid would slowly empty. Ouch, I thought in my head. That looks like it hurts.

Even though my grandma has had many surgeries and other rough patches in her life, she still persevered through all the tough times and I think that's awesome. "Look at that sunset," my grandma whispers as she pulls a black Nikon camera out of her big overflowing purse.

She snaps a perfect picture of the pink, blue and purple sky. The birds in the background are perfectly flying above the orange sun. The leaves of the palm trees leave a silhouette of their shape shadowing the sky. As she goes through all of her pictures on her memory, I look in awe at all the amazing photos she has taken on the camera.

My grandma is as creative as a mom on Pinterest. Not only does she love photography, but she loves acting, directing, and basically the entire theatre as a whole. She always tells me stories about when she was in the theatre and how much she loved directing the play, *The Musical Comedy Murders of 1940*. She has a long association with the Civic and absolutely loves it. My grandma is very talented and creative and I think it's awesome how devoted and dedicated she is to the arts.

My grandma is so very important to me. I haven't spent as much time with her as I would like to, but I'm glad I can still see her the amount of time I can. She is so positive and cheerful when things aren't going well. She is so strong after having medical issues and she is so creative and devoted to the things she loves. She is the best grandmother a granddaughter could ever ask for. I am so happy to have a grandma that will always love and care for me.

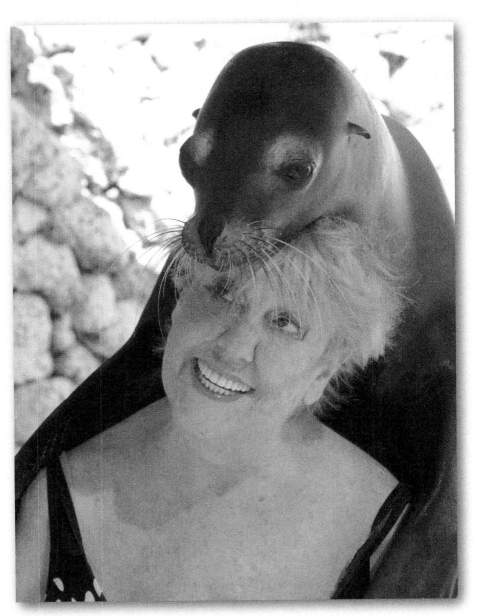

Meeting the sea lion in Nassau.

Chapter 20
AFTER THE FALL

I am writing this in 2017, which started off as a good year. The previous November, our little family vacationed in St. Martin and we had a blast. I even drove a jet ski. The local water sports business provided a way to protect my oxygen from getting wet. Our guide, Johnathan, was informative and funny. In January, we rented a condo on Anna Maria Island from my wonderful niece, Bridget. It was our first time in that part of Florida so we stayed for two weeks. The first week we explored the island by ourselves. The second week Rosemary and Alan joined us. We discovered great restaurants including The Feast and The Chart House. We had dined at the Phoenix Chart House for a couple of anniversaries and loved the salad bar which included caviar.

February found us in the Bahamas for our anniversary/get away from the Michigan weather trip. Because of a SNAFU with our room, we were upgraded to the penthouse suite. And it was sweet. Marble floors and a 180° view of the bay. It offered one huge bathroom which included a Jacuzzi tub, a walk-in shower, terry cloth bathrobes and slippers. There was a half-bath off of the living area. The bedroom provided a king-size, four-poster bed with lush sheets and pillows. They gifted us with delicious chocolate covered strawberries. In addition, the staff gave us a $40 voucher to use at the beach bar. We were thankful for the SNAFU as we basked on the sun beds by the pool. On a boating excursion to Dolphin Encounters, I was kissed by a sea lion.

March came in like a shattered lamb. I felt run down with no energy whatsoever. It was difficult to get up off of the couch. In previous visits, Dr. Chan had suggested I be tested for sleep apnea, [+12] but I procrastinated because I didn't want another medical contraption to deal with. After he convinced me I would feel better, I went to the clinic and was wired up. Anyone who has endured these sleep tests will confirm that you just don't sleep. You can't move because of the connections on your body and the mask is tight and binding. I wasn't able to tolerate it and I felt as though I was suffocating. However, the results came back to reveal I had paused or stopped breathing twenty-three times an hour. With another appointment, the sleep staff found a mask that fit semi-comfortably, so I now put on the elephant tubing along with the oxygen. The first couple of nights were unpleasant, but after a couple of weeks I learned to accept it. My sleep apnea number dropped dramatically from twenty-three to .01 times an hour.

Still exhausted in May, I went to U of M for my regular checkup and a blood draw revealed my red count was very low at 7.4. For women, a normal count should be between 12 to 15. No wonder I was feeling run down. Dr. Chan and Ros wanted to check me into the hospital immediately for a blood transfusion. I didn't want to be in Ann Arbor again, so much to their dismay, I declined. Rich and I bargained with them and came up with a solution. I promised I would go to our local hospital the first thing in the morning for another blood draw. If the numbers were up, great, no need to proceed. However, if the numbers were down, I would have the transfusion done at Bronson. I'm certain Dr. Chan wasn't happy with that idea, but he finally agreed. However, he made a stipulation that I was to make an appointment with a nephrologist in Kalamazoo.

I have so much respect for Dr. Chan and Ros. They have been with me from the very beginning. They understand my frustrations, so they are often lenient with certain situations. I appreciate them so much.

I went to Bronson the next day for another blood draw and the results were higher; 8.9, but not high enough. Rich found a nephrologist, Dr. "L", close by and we made our first appointment. When we met him, he revealed he had seen me in 2010, but I didn't remember. I'd seen so many doctors by then.

With formalities aside, Dr. "L" ultimately dropped the big bomb. He informed me, that besides having anemia, I was in stage four kidney failure.

He went on to discuss dialysis and all that goes with the process. He wanted to know if I would be interested in a study for a new drug for anemia that was **NOT** FDA approved. However, there was an approved anemia shot if I wanted that option. He was very informative by explaining "fistulas" and other medical Greek that neither Rich nor I understood.

All I heard was dialysis and my brain shut down. I can't even begin to describe how I felt. I needed time to process the new information because I was on overload. A raging alarm bell was going off in my head distracting my concentration. I finally had to tell him I couldn't comprehend any more facts. For the past ten years I had been dealing with medical issues and I've been able to cope, somewhat. But this was SERIOUS S**T. Not that what I've been through wasn't serious, but to me, this was a death sentence. I was so shocked that this was in my future. The way he continued to talk, he meant the <u>near</u> future. He was implying I should make an appointment right then and there to go forward.

With any medical situation, before I agreed to anything, whether a procedure, or medication, I always discussed it with Dr. Chan and Ros. When we arrived home, I called them immediately. I wanted them to know the details of the appointment. I needed some definition of what happened because I was terrified. Oh, and regarding the study, I had already determined, no f****** way.

"We didn't mean to scare you," Ros said. "We just wanted to let you know this could happen in the future. We have many lung transplant patients who are in the same situation as you and have survived for a long time.

So, it was decided I would receive the "safe" anemia shot to see if it improved my lack of energy. If the results weren't to my satisfaction, we would decide where to go from there. I've proved them to be wrong on so many occasions, maybe this was just another bump in the road.

I saw this quote on Facebook: "*I don't know how my story will end, but nowhere will it ever read . . . "I gave up."* I wish I could say that. I've always believed I would make it through whatever was thrown at me. That's probably why I've survived so long. "*That which does not kill us, makes us stronger?*" I wish I could say, "Spending four hours a day, three days a week in the hospital on dialysis with another operation to place the fistula – no problem, let's do it." I already go once a month for an IV, which I call a booster shot of immuno-suppressants. What's another day? I wish I could say that, but quite frankly, I've had enough. It was not an option for me to spend more time in the hospital. If this is going to reduce my quality of life, I'm done. I want to live, not just survive. When I expressed these feelings to Rich, he was extremely disheartened. He told me that in 2012, after the rejection episode, he promised himself he would do anything to keep me alive. But it's not in our hands. It never was.

However, after three months of anemia shots, my count is up to 9.4. After four months using the C-Pap, I'm sleeping better, at least seven hours a night. And I have a little more energy. On September 30, 2017, I did a walk-on role in *Young Frankenstein* for the Kalamazoo Civic. It was a wonderful night. I concluded I hadn't been on Mainstage in 20 years. Everyone in the cast and on the crew were so welcoming and encouraging, and I had a blast! The stage manager, a longtime friend, looked the other way when

I stayed on longer than initially suggested. In the opening number, when the cast began to dance, I grabbed my back-side and hobbled over to the stage right wall and hung there until they were done. Got a HUGE laugh! I even took part in the curtain call. What a night! The proverb is true: There's no people like show people.

So, for now, "*I'll* <u>will</u> *See You Later*, Dad." Much later.

APPLAUSE

. . . goes out to the producers of my script. Without their patience, love and dedication, I would not be here today: Rich, my wonderful husband and knight in shining armor. You've gone above and beyond the call. You kept me going when I wanted to give up. You made me laugh at the most serious situations. You are an inspiration.

My beautiful and loving daughter Susan, I'm so proud of you. I love your sense of humor amid chaos. You may have been frightened on the inside, but not wanting to upset me, you remained stoic amidst the storm and I love you for that.

To my sister and my hero Rosemary, who always seems to rescue me when I'm in distress. I'm so glad you and Alan moved to Kalamazoo so we can share more memories. I love how all four of us click and have fun and enjoy life.

Thanks to my brother in law, Alan, for his quick wit and guidance which were non-stop. I adore you. I couldn't ask for a better friend.

To my beautiful granddaughter Hannah, with your positive attitude and intellect you will have a wonderful life. Remember to keep smiling in life and use, "no biggy" whenever you can.

Aaron, who brought happiness to our daughter's life, I will always adore you for that. You are a great addition to our family. I love your laisser-faire attitude, and your knowledge in all things.

. . . to the technicians, the people behind the scenes. You don't see them, but without them, the show wouldn't go on. Dr. Kevin Chan, Ros, Dr. Shay, Dr. Pickens, University of Michigan Hospital staff, Bronson Hospital staff, Gift of Life Michigan, Bronson Health Club.

. . . for my script readers who kept me on the right track: Wilma Kahn, Leeanne Seaver, Deb Hanley, Bev Riley, Laura B. Wilbur, Kitty Kachniewicz, Glyni Fenn, Kathleen Weissert, Susan Hanselman and Bernie Brommel.

Special applause to those who donated their insightfulness to my story: James Carver, Terri Pelfernese, John Shea, Terry Johnston, Laura Higgins Kohlar, Dr. William H. Fenn P.A.-C; PhD, and Dan Fleischaker.

And the many guest stars who made the production possible: Janet Gover, Catherine Batts, Brenda O'Rourke, Bridget O'Ryan, Ginny Bach and the whole Jaws and Joints team. Jean Compere and the Heavy Breathers, Randi Keck, Art and Linda Nemitz, Erwan and Cyril Jesson-Ripoll, and last but not least, Kathy Anderson and Jack Prichard for many Euchre games and dinners when I wasn't able to do anything else.

I also want to acknowledge the Kalamazoo Civic Theatre for giving me my life and my passion.

Love to all~

CLUE THE MUSICAL
Glossary

[+1] Alpha-1 Antitrypsin Deficiency (AAT) is an inherited condition that raises your risk for lung and liver disease. Alpha-1 antitrypsin (AAT) is a protein that protects the lungs. The liver makes it. If the AAT proteins aren't the right shape, they get stuck in the liver cells and can't reach the lungs.

Symptoms of AAT deficiency include: Shortness of breath and wheezing, Repeated lung infections, Tiredness, Rapid heartbeat upon standing, Vision problems, and Weight loss.

[+2] Lawrence Stebenne obit.txt - Clark County NV Archives Obituaries - August 1918

"A. J. Stebenne, Democratic nominee for the office of district attorney, returned last Wednesday from his visit to Denver, Colorado, where he was called by the accidental death of his brother, Larry. Larry Stebenne was employed by the Denver Tramway Company as a painting foreman, and had been called to a sub-plant to inspect some work that had been finished by one of his men, and while in the act of descending from the roof of the building, he accidentally touched his arm against a wire carrying 13,000 volts, which was running along parallel to the top of the roof. He lived fourteen hours after receiving the injury. Mr. Stebenne's death will be extremely felt by his fellow working men, for it was Larry who, after being in the employment of the company but four months had caused the consolidation of several labor organizations, which had in the past, had received no recognition from the company, and it was Larry who, after being elected chairman of a committee to visit the company on behalf of the brotherhood in an endeavor to secure the signature of the company for a closed shop. On the night, just before he met his death, and after a two-hour session, he was successful in securing the signature of the company to an agreement recognizing the labor union and doing away with the open shop, which had been the policy of the company for many years. Labor lost a valuable member in the death of Larry Stebenne."

[+3] Coldwater Regional Mental Health Center was opened on May 21, 1874. Once admitted, children participated in "family-like" life in cottages and a placing-out program. Children learned reading, spelling, counting, calisthenics, singing, ciphering and slate drawing. By the turn of the century, the facility had become the only home in Michigan admitting both normal and handicapped children.

In 1939, the Children's Village became the Coldwater State Home & Training School, and persons of all ages with more serious handicaps were admitted. By 1960, there were 2,900 residents. During the 1970s, special education, training, and living experiences in communities reduced the number of residents to fewer than 700. Renamed the Coldwater Regional Center of Developmental Disabilities in 1978, the remodeled facility provided training programs for independent living and self-help. In 1985, the center converted to a psychiatric hospital, and in 1986, its name changed to the Coldwater Regional Mental Health Center. It closed in June 1992.

[+4] Camille was formed on August 14, 1969 and dissipated August 22. The winds reached 175 mph. There were 259 fatalities and damages reached $1.42 billion.

[+5] Part of the culture here since 1929, the Kalamazoo Civic is one of the fifth largest theatres in the country. Dorothy Dalton, daughter of William E. Upjohn, of pharmaceutical claim, wanted to pursue a theatre career in New York City. Her parents, especially her father, were opposed and wanted her to stay home. He promised to build her a theatre if she complied. And so, the Civic was built, and what a theatre it is. The tin roof and the front of the building were designed to resemble a circus tent. The carvings around the doorways give the impression of tent flaps. You'll find the style continues throughout the building with replicas of circus wagon escutcheons adorning the spiral staircase and four large murals depicting a circus and a traveling show grace the walls of the Green Room.

There are two additional performance spaces across the street from the main auditorium – The Carver Center, named for Norman and Louise Carver who were part of the founding group with Dorothy Dalton. And the Suzanne D. Parish Theatre, named for Dalton's daughter.

In 1958 James Carver, Norman's son, was hired as production manager and promoted to Managing Director in 1974. He retired in 1997 and Steven Carver, Jim's son, took over the lead position in 2016 with interim directors in between.

[+6] Labor was a prominent power in 1981. When the air traffic controllers went out on strike, the labor movement was still seen as a central force in American government and politics. Both parties, Republican and Democrat, saw labor that way.

It was an important moment in American history because Ronald Reagan was in the first months of his presidency and he was in the middle of rolling out the Reagan revolution. He wanted to reorganize the relationship between government and the labor movement.

The PATCO (Professional Air Traffic Controllers) strike happened at this important turning point in American history, and it left a very profound legacy. Reagan threatened those strikers to return to work within 48 hours of their walkout, and when they refused, he not only fired them, but permanently replaced them. With that action, he sent a message that many employers even in the private sector acted upon after that. Many believe Reagan acted in the hopes of stifling 46,000 postal workers from striking as their contract was due shortly after PATCO.

Hitchhiker's Guide to the Galaxy.

[+7] The State Theatre has been a fixture in downtown Kalamazoo since 1927. The original founder of the theatre was Colonel William Butterfield with John Eberson as the designer. The early roots of the theatre were founded in Vaudeville featuring opera, dramas, big bands, ballet, dance reviews, stage shows, and movies.

The theatre was renovated in 1964 to remove the original theatre sign which was beginning to deteriorate. These renovations changed some of the original ornate look and feel of the theatre, but enabled it to continue operating until 1982 when W.S. Butterfield Theatre Inc. decided to close the landmark.

[+8] The Kalamazoo Promise. . .

- is for ALL students of the Kalamazoo Public Schools (KPS).
- You must reside within the boundaries of KPS.
- You must have at least all of the high school years (9-12) in KPS (enrollment & residency) and graduate from KPS (Central / Loy Norrix/ Phoenix).
- The Kalamazoo Promise will not end. It is set up to go on for many years to come.
- The Kalamazoo Promise is a 4-year scholarship (a bachelor degree or 130 credits, whichever occurs first).
- You have ten years from the time you graduate from high school to use your Promise and can start and stop any time.
- The Kalamazoo Promise covers tuition and mandatory fees.
- Students sign up for The Kalamazoo Promise at the beginning of their senior year. Meetings are held for all seniors each fall. There are two simple forms to fill out for The Kalamazoo Promise.

- There is an appeal process for students during their senior year, especially for hardship cases (e.g., custody, death in the family, and foster care placement).
- All students using The Kalamazoo Promise at KVCC may attend part-time.

[+9] An oxygen concentrator (also sometimes called "oxygen generator") is a medical device used to deliver oxygen to those who require it. People may require it if they have a condition that causes or results in low levels of oxygen in their blood. These oxygen concentrators are normally obtained via prescription and therefore cannot be purchased over the counter. Oxygen concentrators are powered by plugging in to an electrical outlet or by battery. If the concentrator is powered by an electric battery, that battery will need to be charged by plugging into an outlet. Several parts make up a concentrator, including a compressor, sieve bed filter, and circuit boards.

An oxygen concentrator has a compressing element, but it should not be confused with compressed oxygen or an oxygen tank. Whereas a tank has a set amount of oxygen that it dispenses, a concentrator filters in air, compresses it, and delivers air continuously. The air supply will never run out. Instead of refilling compressed air, the concentrator just needs access to power.

HOW DOES AN OXYGEN CONCENTRATOR WORK?
An oxygen concentrator works much like a window air conditioning unit: it takes in air, modifies it and delivers it in a new form. An oxygen concentrator takes in air and purifies it for use by people requiring medical oxygen due to low oxygen levels in their blood.

It works by:

- Taking in air from its surroundings
- Compressing air, while the cooling mechanism keeps the concentrator from overheating
- Removing nitrogen from the air via filter and sieve beds

- Adjusting delivery settings with an electronic interface
- Delivering the purified oxygen via a nasal cannula or mask

[+10] Spirometry is used to assess how well your lungs work by measuring how much air you inhale; how much you exhale and how quickly you exhale. Spirometry is used to diagnose asthma, chronic obstructive pulmonary disease (COPD) and other conditions that affect breathing.

[+11] Cushingoid: Having the constellation of symptoms and signs caused by an excess of cortisol hormone: that is, Cushing syndrome. While facial puffiness and weight gain are typical features of a Cushingoid appearance, Cushing Syndrome is an extremely complex hormonal condition that involves many areas of the body.

[+12] Sleep apnea occurs when you regularly stop breathing for ten seconds or longer during sleep. It can be mild, moderate, or severe, depending on the number of times in an hour that your breathing stops (apnea) or becomes very shallow (hypopnea). Apnea episodes may occur from five to one hundred times an hour.

NEWSIES
Updates.

- In the late 1980's my brother and I had a falling out and we lost communication only to reconnect in 2003. However, a few years later, the bridge crumbled again. I saw him at a family Christmas party in 2016, and a funeral in 2017, but the bridge is too difficult to repair.
- I haven't seen my sister Nyoda since my rejection in 2012. She has moved to assisted living facilities with questionable sanitary conditions, and I can't afford to compromise my health. I understand there are germs everywhere, but they seem elevated in these situations.
- Earlier in our marriage, we only saw Rich's brother on holidays when we were in Chicago. He was moving around the country for his career, but we never ended up in the same place. Eventually, whatever reason, he broke off all contact and we didn't hear from him for 15 years.

   In 2009, he reconnected and stayed with us for a few months after a devastating life event. In 2016, still living in New York, he suffered two strokes. Rich visits often, but it is difficult to maintain communication given the distance and his state of mind.
- After many setbacks in the early stages of recovery, I really didn't think I was going to live. I decided I wanted to contact people who had made an impact on my life. In 2009 I connected with old friends, teachers and yes, my old boyfriend. We continue to email, and chat every once in a while. I've only seen him once when I went to his mother's visitation. (I adored his mother.) He has a lovely wife and appears to be happy. I've never told him thank you for dumping me! With his actions I met my soul mate and my hero, Rich. Maybe he'll buy my book and read it himself!
- Susan was divorced in 2013. 'nuff said.

ABOUT THE AUTHOR

Ten years after her double lung transplant, Cathie Higgins Weir is now a charter member of the Heavy Breathers Club. She and her husband Rich reside in Kalamazoo, MI and have been married for 47 years . . . 40 happily.

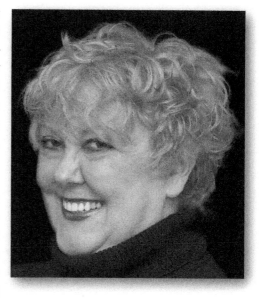

As a result of her 30-year career in theatre Rich proclaims, "I never know what character I'll wake up to in the morning!" He was extremely anxious when Cathie played Lady Macbeth. Their passion is traveling, especially to tropical destinations with their daughter Susan, her beau Aaron and granddaughter Hannah. But their rescue Cairn Terrier, "Scary Kerry" stays behind at the doggie hotel. Besides theatre and traveling, Cathie loves swimming, water aerobics and taking long naps.

Made in the USA
Middletown, DE
14 November 2018